PUBLIC HEALTH IN THE 21ST CENTURY

GLOBAL MALARIA THREAT AND THE U.S. RESPONSE

PUBLIC HEALTH IN THE 21ST CENTURY

Additional books in this series can be found on Nova's website under the Series tab.

Additional E-books in this series can be found on Nova's website under the E-books tab.

PUBLIC HEALTH IN THE 21ST CENTURY

GLOBAL MALARIA THREAT AND THE U.S. RESPONSE

ROBERT N. MOYNIHAN
EDITOR

Nova Science Publishers, Inc.
New York

For permission to use material from this book please contact us:
Telephone 631-231-7269; Fax 631-231-8175
Web Site: http://www.novapublishers.com

Additional color graphics may be available in the e-book version of this book.

Library of Congress Cataloging-in-Publication Data

Global malaria threat and the U.S. response / editor, Robert N. Moynihan.
p. ; cm. Includes index.
ISBN 978-1-61324-572-9 (hardcover)
1. Malaria--Prevention--Africa South of the Sahara. 2. Malaria--Prevention--United States. 3. Malaria--Prevention--International cooperation 4. United States. Tom Lantos and Henry J. Hyde United States Global Leadership against HIV/AIDS, Tuberculosis, and Malaria Reauthorization Act of 2008. I. Moynihan, Robert N.
[DNLM: 1. United States. Tom Lantos and Henry J. Hyde United States Global Leadership against HIV/AIDS, Tuberculosis, and Malaria Reauthorization Act of 2008. 2. United States. Agency for International Development. 3. Malaria--prevention & control--Africa South of the Sahara. 4. Malaria--prevention & control--United States. 5. International Cooperation--Africa South of the Sahara. 6. International Cooperation--United States. 7. World Health--Africa South of the Sahara. 8. World Health--United States. WC 765]
RA644.M2G56 2011 362.196'9362--dc23

2011014537

Published by Nova Science Publishers, Inc. + New York

CONTENTS

PREFACE

In 2009, malaria infected an estimated 225 million people and killed 781,000 people, most of whom, were children under the age of five in sub-Saharan Africa. Despite the current burden of disease, malaria is preventable and treatable. Congress has increasingly recognized malaria as an important foreign policy issue, and the United States has become a major player in the global response to the disease. The 112th Congress will likely debate the appropriate funding levels and optimum strategy for addressing the continued challenge of global malaria. This book outlines basic facts related to global malaria, including characteristics of the epidemic and U.S. legislation, programs, funding and partnerships related to the global response to malaria.

Chapter 1- In 2009, malaria infected an estimated 225 million people and killed 781,000 people, most of whom were children under the age of five in sub-Saharan Africa. Despite the current burden of disease, malaria is preventable and treatable. Congress has increasingly recognized malaria as an important foreign policy issue, and the United States has become a major player in the global response to the disease. The 112th Congress will likely debate the appropriate funding levels and optimum strategy for addressing the continued challenge of global malaria.

Chapter 2- Malaria prevention and control is a major U.S. foreign assistance objective and is a core component of a comprehensive U.S. Government (USG) Global Health Initiative (GHI), announced in May 2009 by President Barack Obama to reduce the burden of disease and strengthen communities around the world. The 2008 Tom Lantos and Henry J. Hyde Global Leadership against HIV/AIDS, Tuberculosis, and Malaria Act (Lantos/Hyde Act) authorizes up to $5 billion in USG funding for malaria prevention and control for the period FY2009–2013. This Act calls for the development of a comprehensive, multiyear USG strategy to combat malaria globally and strengthen the capacity of the United States to be an effective leader of international efforts to reduce the burden of malaria.

Chapter 3- This report outlines the U.S. Government's (USG's) contributions to a dramatic scale-up of malaria prevention and treatment measuresacross 15 President's Malaria Initiative (PMI)-supported countries over the past four years. Many of these countries have reportedsignificant reductions in under-five mortality, and there is strong and growing evidence that malaria prevention and treatment effortsare a major factor in these reductions. Throughout this report, we highlight the USG's role in the scale-up of malaria interventions,training of health workers, support for services and commodities, and health systems strengthening. Progress in malaria control is aresult of the collective actions of African governments; international donors, including the USG, The Global Fund to Fight AIDS,Tuberculosis and Malaria (Global Fund), and World Bank; and nongovernmental organizations.

In: Global Malaria Threat and the U.S. Response ISBN: 978-1-61324-572-9
Editor: Robert N. Moynihan

Chapter 1

U.S. RESPONSE TO THE GLOBAL THREAT OF MALARIA: BASIC FACTS

Alexandra E. Kendall

SUMMARY

In 2009, malaria infected an estimated 225 million people and killed 781,000 people, most of whom were children under the age of five in sub-Saharan Africa. Despite the current burden of disease, malaria is preventable and treatable. Congress has increasingly recognized malaria as an important foreign policy issue, and the United States has become a major player in the global response to the disease. The 112th Congress will likely debate the appropriate funding levels and optimum strategy for addressing the continued challenge of global malaria.

Congress has enacted several key pieces of legislation related to global malaria control. These include the Assistance for International Malaria Control Act of 2000 (P.L. 106-570); the U.S. Leadership Against HIV/AIDS, Tuberculosis, and Malaria Act of 2003 (P.L. 108-25); and the Tom Lantos and Henry J. Hyde United States Global Leadership Against HIV/AIDS, Tuberculosis, and Malaria Reauthorization Act of 2008 (P.L. 110-293). These acts have authorized funds to be used in the fights against malaria and have shaped the ways in which U.S. malaria programs are coordinated and managed, including through the creation of the U.S. Global Malaria

Coordinator at the United States Agency for International Development (USAID).

In 2005, in response to growing international calls for global malaria control and to the success of the President's Emergency Plan for AIDS Relief (PEPFAR), President George W. Bush launched the President's Malaria Initiative (PMI), which aims to halve the burden of malaria morbidity and mortality in 70% of at-risk populations in sub-Saharan Africa by 2014. PMI brought significant new attention and funding to U.S. malaria programs and made the United States one of the largest donors for malaria efforts. While U.S. funding for global malaria programs has increased each fiscal year since FY2004, support for malaria interventions increased most precipitously beginning in FY2007 as PMI has expanded into new countries. President Obama has continued to support PMI and has called for greater spending on malaria programs in each of his budget requests. The President's FY20 12 budget requests $691 million for global malaria efforts.

There is evidence that the growing international response to malaria has had some success in controlling the epidemic. Since 2000, 11 African countries have experienced at least a 50% reduction in either confirmed malaria cases or malaria admissions and deaths. The decreases in each of these African countries are associated with intense malaria control activities. Despite these successes, several key issues pose challenges to effective scale-up of the response to malaria. First, increasing reports of drug-resistant malaria in Asia and insecticide-resistant mosquitoes in Africa threaten the success of malaria control programs. Second, weak health systems, including shortages in health care personnel and inadequate supply chain networks, have limited the delivery of essential commodities for malaria control. There is also debate within the global health community over whether malaria efforts should increasingly target areas where malaria elimination is possible or whether efforts should remain concentrated on malaria control.

This report outlines basic facts related to global malaria, including characteristics of the epidemic and U.S. legislation, programs, funding, and partnerships related to the global response to malaria.

INTRODUCTION

The United States has supported anti-malaria programs since the 1950s. Global malaria received greater attention in 2005 when President Bush launched the President's Malaria Initiative (PMI), a five-year plan to expand

U.S. malaria efforts. In FY2008, Congress significantly increased its funding for global malaria and authorized the creation of the U.S. Global Malaria Coordinator at the United States Agency for International Development (USAID) to oversee all U.S. malaria efforts. President Barack Obama has emphasized combating malaria in his Global Health Initiative (GHI) and has called for increasing funding for these efforts. This report provides background information on malaria and explains the key components of the U.S. response.

DESCRIPTION OF MALARIA

Malaria is an infectious disease that is transmitted to people through the bite of infected mosquitoes. The disease infects red blood cells, causing a range of symptoms that include fever, headache, and vomiting. Although malaria is preventable and curable, if left untreated, it can be fatal. Young children, pregnant women, and individuals with HIV/AIDS are particularly vulnerable to malaria due to their weakened immune systems.

GLOBAL MALARIA STATISTICS[1]

Malaria Cases: The World Health Organization (WHO) estimates that half of the world's population is at risk of malaria infection. Malaria is prevalent in 106 countries, referred to as malaria-endemic countries. In 2009, there were approximately 225 million cases of malaria worldwide, down from approximately 233 cases in 2000. Since 2000, 32 countries outside of Africa have experienced more than a 50% reduction in reported malaria cases, and 11 African countries have experienced at least a 50% reduction in either confirmed malaria cases or malaria admissions and deaths.

Malaria Deaths: The malaria death toll declined from 985,000 in 2000 to 781,000 people in 2009. Roughly 85% of 2009 malaria-related deaths occurred among children younger than five.

REGIONAL DISTRIBUTION OF MALARIA[2]

Malaria occurs worldwide, though it is heavily concentrated in what are categorized by WHO as the African, South-East Asian, and the Eastern Mediterranean regions (Figure 1).[3]

- In 2009, about 78% of all malaria cases and 91% of all malaria-related deaths occurred in the WHO Africa region. There are 43 malaria-endemic countries in the Africa region.
- The WHO South-East Asia region was home to 15% of all malaria cases and 6% of malaria-related deaths in 2009. Of the 10 malaria-endemic countries in the South-East Asia region, India, Bangladesh, Indonesia, and Myanmar (Burma) make up 97% of all malaria cases.
- The WHO Eastern Mediterranean region was home to 5% of all malaria cases and 2% of malaria-related deaths in 2009. Of the region's 12 malaria-endemic countries, Afghanistan, Pakistan, Somalia, and Sudan make up 90% of malaria cases.

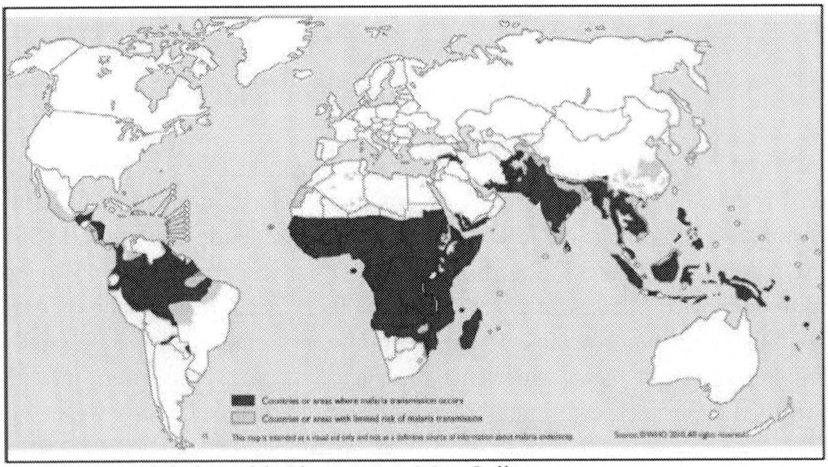

Source: WHO, *Global Health Observatory,* Map Gallery, httpi/gamapserver.who.int/mapLibrary/.

Notes: Countries or areas in dark blue are where malaria transmission occurs. Countries or areas in light blue are those with limited risk of malaria transmission.

Figure 1. Malaria, Countries or Areas at Risk of Transmission, 2009.

Malaria Prevention and Treatment

The international community applies four strategies for combating malaria:

Treatment: Anti-malarial treatments include chloroquine, primaquine, and artesmisinin-based combination therapy (ACT). ACT is the preferred treatment in areas with particularly deadly forms of malaria or with drug resistance to earlier generations of anti-malarials. Multi-drug resistant malaria is found worldwide, and there is evidence that ACT resistance is occurring in Asia.

Intermittent Preventive Treatment in Pregnancy (IPTp): In areas with high concentrations of malaria, physicians give pregnant women an anti-malarial drug to prevent them from transmitting the disease to their infants.

Insecticide-Treated Bed Nets (ITNs): Insecticides used to treat bed nets kill and repel mosquitoes. ITNs are used as personal protection against mosquito bites, but evidence suggests that high community coverage of ITNs can lower the number of mosquitoes in a general area and reduce the life span of mosquitoes that remain. ITNs retain effective levels of insecticide for up to six months. Newly developed long-lasting insecticide-treated nets (LLINs) last for at least three years.

Indoor Residual Spraying (IRS): IRS involves covering household walls with an insecticide to kill any mosquito that comes into contact with the surfaces for several months. To be effective, IRS must be applied to a high percentage (80%) of household surfaces. Resistance to insecticides is a growing concern.

While there is presently no malaria vaccine, research is ongoing. There are currently over a dozen vaccine candidates in clinical development, and one, produced by GlaxoSmithKline, is in clinical trials.

Key U.S. Legislation on Global Malaria

- On December 27, 2000, President Bill Clinton signed into law the Assistance for International Malaria Control Act (P.L. 106-570). The act authorized $50 million per year for FY200 1 and FY2002 for anti-malaria activities in countries with high malaria prevalence.

- On May 27, 2003, President George W. Bush signed into law the United States Leadership Against HIV/AIDS, Tuberculosis, and Malaria Act of 2003 (Leadership Act, P.L. 108-25). The act authorized $15 billion for global HIV/AIDS, TB, and malaria programs from FY2004 through FY2008. The act recognized malaria control as a major foreign policy objective, though it did not specify an amount for bilateral malaria programs.
  The act also prohibited U.S. contributions to the Global Fund to Fight AIDS, Tuberculosis and Malaria (Global Fund) (See "Key Partners in the Response to Global Malaria") from exceeding 33% of funds contributed from all sources.
- On July 24, 2008, President Bush signed into law the Tom Lantos and Henry J. Hyde U.S. Global Leadership Against HIV/AIDS, Tuberculosis, and Malaria Reauthorization Act of 2008 (Lantos-Hyde Act, P.L. 110-293). The act authorized $48 billion for global HIV/AIDS, TB, and malaria programs from FY2008 through FY2013, including $5 billion for malaria programs over five years.
  The act also created the position of U.S. Global Malaria Coordinator at USAID. The Malaria Coordinator is charged with overseeing all U.S. anti-malaria efforts, submitting an annual report to Congress describing U.S. malaria programs, and developing a five- year strategic plan for U.S. efforts to combat malaria.

U.S. GLOBAL MALARIA PROGRAMS

The United States has supported global malaria control efforts since the 1950s. Efforts to expand U.S. malaria programs and improve their coordination increased following the announcement of the President's Malaria Initiative (PMI) in 2005. PMI represented a growing acknowledgement of the efficacy of malaria prevention and treatment strategies and built on the success of the President's Emergency Plan for AIDS Relief (PEPFAR) in harnessing resources to combat a disease. PMI was initially created as a five-year, $1.2 billion effort to increase U.S. engagement in global malaria control and reduce malaria-related deaths by 50% in 15 high-burden focus countries. Focus countries were selected according to several criteria, including high malaria burden, capacity to implement anti-malaria programs, and willingness to partner with the United States. PMI has since expanded into two other malaria-endemic countries in Africa (Table 1).

PMI is an interagency initiative run by USAID and jointly implemented by USAID and the Centers for Disease Control and Prevention (CDC). The U.S. Global Malaria Coordinator at USAID coordinates malaria efforts across a number of agencies and departments, including CDC, the Department of Defense (DOD), and the National Institutes of Health (NIH). Oversight duties are shared with an Interagency Steering Group composed of representatives from USAID, CDC/the Department of Health and Human Services (HHS), the Department of State, DOD, the National Security Council, and the Office of Management and Budget. USAID and CDC also provide bilateral malaria assistance to a handful of countries not designated as PMI focus countries. Figure 2 depicts all countries that receive U.S. bilateral malaria assistance.

Table 1. PMI Focus Countries.

The PMI Focus Countries have been added over the course of several fiscal years:
FY2006: Angola, Tanzania, Uganda
FY2007: Malawi, Mozambique, Rwanda, Senegal
FY2008: Benin, Ethiopia, Ghana, Kenya, Liberia, Madagascar, Mali, Zambia
FY2011: Nigeria, Democratic Republic of the Congo

Note: PMI countries selected in FY2006, FY2007, and FY2008 represent the original 15 PMI focus countries.

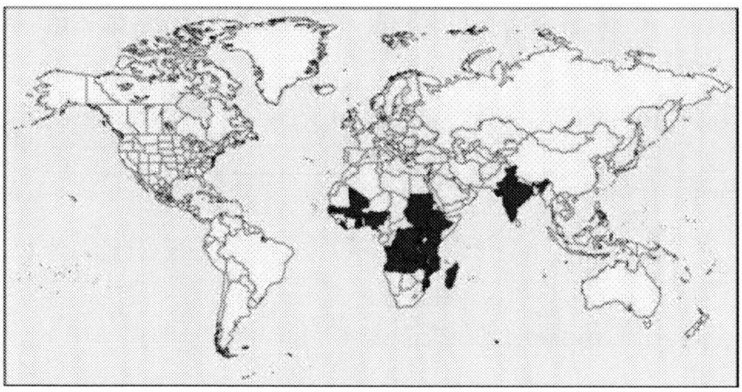

Source: Kaiser Family Foundation, September 2010, http://facts.kff.org/chart.aspx?ch=876.

Notes: Countries in blue are those selected to receive U.S. bilateral support for malaria according to the Department of State FY2011 Foreign Operations Congressional Budget Justification. Countries in yellow do not receive U.S. bilateral support for malaria.

Figure 2. U.S. Bilateral Malaria Programs.

President Obama has indicated support for an expanded U.S. malaria program. On May 5, 2009, the President announced the six-year, $63 billion Global Health Initiative (GHI), a new effort to develop a comprehensive U.S. global health strategy. Malaria is one of the GHI's six priority areas, and PMI is considered a key component of the GHI, reflecting the Administration's belief that scaled-up malaria interventions can help maximize health impact per dollar spent. The GHI calls for a more integrated U.S. response to global health issues, including better coordination between malaria and maternal and child health programs. The GHI also calls for a shift in U.S. global health strategy from one focused on specific diseases to a more comprehensive approach to health, including a focus on health system strengthening.

In April 2010, in response to congressional reporting requirements to develop a coordinated approach to global malaria, USAID, HHS (including CDC), and the Department of State released a joint "Lantos-Hyde United States Government Malaria Strategy."[4] The strategy explains how U.S. malaria programs will advance the goals of the GHI and outlines key targets for the U.S. malaria program from 2009 to 2014. Key goals include the following:

- halve the burden of malaria (morbidity and mortality) in 70% of at-risk populations in sub-Saharan Africa;
- limit the spread of anti-malarial multi-drug resistance in Southeast Asia and the Americas;
- assist host countries to revise and update their National Malaria Control Strategies and Plans to reflect the declining burden of malaria; and
- link U.S. malaria efforts with host country malaria plans.

IMPLEMENTING U.S. AGENCIES

U.S. agencies supporting global malaria control efforts include the following:

- **United States Agency for International Development:** USAID manages PMI programs in the PMI focus countries. USAID also supports malaria control programs in several other countries and facilitates efforts to identify and contain anti-malarial drug resistance through two regional programs in the Amazon Basin and the Mekong

Delta. USAID's malaria programs focus on five key areas: IRS, ITNs, IPTp, diagnosis and treatment, and pesticide management.

- **Centers for Disease Control and Prevention:** CDC jointly implements PMI with USAID. CDC's malaria efforts focus on monitoring and evaluation, disease surveillance, and capacity development for national malaria control programs. CDC also undertakes global malaria research to improve prevention and treatment efforts with an emphasis on LLINs, IRS, and IPTp, and the elimination of malaria.
- **Department of Defense:** DOD supports malaria research, including anti-malaria treatment and vaccine development. Research is conducted at the U.S. Military Malaria Vaccine Program at the Walter Reed Army Institute of Research and the Malaria Research Department at the Navy Medical Research Center.
- **National Institutes of Health:** The National Institute of Allergy and Infectious Diseases (NIAID) of the NIH is the lead U.S. agency supporting malaria research. NIAID works on developing tools for malaria prevention, treatment and control, and enhancing research infrastructure in malaria-endemic countries.

U.S. Global Malaria Assistance Funds

Congress designates funds for malaria to USAID, through State-Foreign Operations appropriations, and to CDC, through Labor, Health and Human Services, and Education appropriations. Congressional appropriations for malaria have consistently increased since FY2004. In response to growing calls within the international community for global malaria control, funding for malaria interventions have increased most precipitously since FY2007 (Table 2 and Figure 3) in support of PMI expansion into new countries. President Obama has continued to support PMI and has called for greater spending on malaria programs in each of his budget requests. The President's FY20 12 budget requests $691 million for global malaria efforts.

Table 2. U.S. Bilateral Funding for Malaria: FY2004-FY20 12 ($ Millions, Current).

Program/ Agency	FY2004 Actual	FY2005 Actual	FY2006 Actual	FY2007 Actual	FY2008 Actual	FY2009 Actual	FY2010 Estimate	FY2004- FY20 10 TOTAL	FY2011 Request	FY2012 Request
USAID Malaria	79.9	90.8	102.0	248.0	349.6	382.5	585.0	1,837.8	680.0	691
Of which, PMI	n/a	4.2	65.5	197.0	295.8	299.9	500.0	1,362.4	600.0	n/s
CDC Malaria	9.2	9.1	9.0	8.9	8.7	9.4	9.4	63.7	9.2	n/s[a]
Malaria Total	89.1	99.9	111.0	256.9	358.3	391.9	594.4	1,901.5	689.2	691

Source: Compiled by CRS from Congressional Budget Justifications, appropriations legislation, and PMI reports.

Notes: "n/a" stands for "not applicable." PMI was established in 2005 and therefore did not receive funding in FY2004. FY2011 Funding is currently provided under a continuing resolution at FY20 10-enacted levels until March 4, 2011.

a. The FY2012 budget request includes $19.6 million for parasitic diseases and malaria. It does not specify an amount for malaria alone, as has been done in previous fiscal years.

Table 3. U.S. Appropriations for the Global Fund: FY2004-FY2012 ($ Millions, Current).

Program/Agency	FY2004 Actual	FY2005 Actual	FY2006 Actual	FY2007 Actual	FY2008 Actual	FY2009 Actual	FY20 10 Estimate	FY 2011 Request	FY20 12 Request
USAID	397.6	248.0	247.5	247.5	0.0	100.0	0.0	0.0	0.0
FY2004 Carryover	-87.8	87.8	n/a	n/a	n/a	n/a	n/a	n/a	n/a
State	0.0	0.0	198.0	377.5	545.5	600.0	750.0	700.0	1,000.0
HHS	149.1	99.2	99.0	99.0	294.8	300.0	300.0	300.0	300.0
Total	458.9	435.0	544.5	724.0	840.3	1,000.0	1,050.0	1,000.0	1,300.0

Source: Compiled by CRS from appropriations legislation.

Notes: In the "FY2004 Carryover" row, "n/a" is used to reflect requirements in the U.S. Leadership Act, which stipulates that U.S. contributions to the Fund not exceed 33% of Fund contributions from all sources. FY2005 Consolidated Appropriations (P.L. 108-447) added this amount to the 2005 contribution, subject to the same 33% limitation.

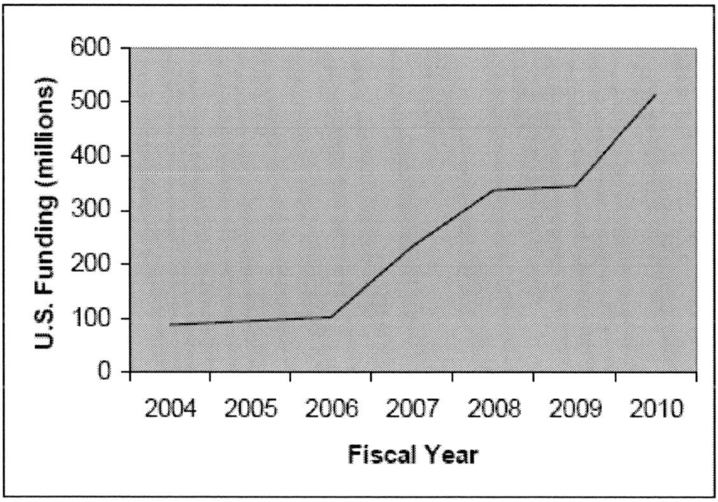

Source: Compiled by CRS from Congressional Budget Justifications.

Figure 3. U.S. Bilateral Funding for Malaria in Constant Dollars: FY2004-FY2010 ($ millions, constant).

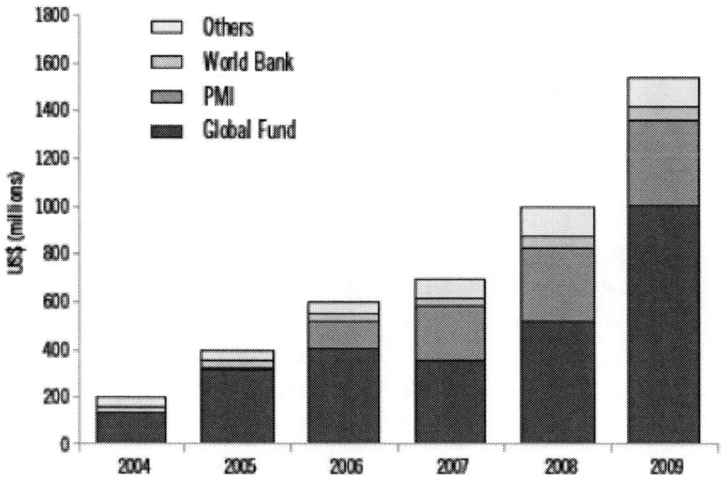

Source: WHO, *World Malaria Report*, 2010, p. 12.

Figure 4. Disbursements to Malaria Endemic Countries from External Donors, 2004-2009.

The United States also supports global malaria programs through contributions to the Global Fund, an international financing mechanism for the response to HIV/AIDS, TB, and malaria. U.S. contributions to the Global Fund support grants for HIV/AIDS, TB, and malaria. The Global Fund has historically directed approximately 25% of its funds for malaria efforts. The United States is the single largest donor to the Global Fund. **Table 3** details actual and proposed U.S. contributions to the Global Fund from FY2004 to FY2012.

The majority of total global funding for malaria control comes from three sources: external donor assistance, national government spending, and household expenditures. According to WHO, of the total malaria spending in 2007, donor assistance accounted for 47%, national government spending accounted for 34%, and household expenditures accounted for 19%.[5] External donor assistance comes primarily from three sources: PMI, the Global Fund, and the World Bank (**Figure 4**). The Global Fund is the single largest donor for malaria efforts. According to the Global Fund, it accounted for 57% of all external financing for malaria in 2008.[6]

Key Partners in the Response to Global Malaria

The United States works with a range of partners to combat malaria, including other national governments, multilateral organizations, non-governmental organizations (NGOs), and the private sector. Key partners include the following:

- **The Global Fund:** The Global Fund was established in 2002 as a public-private partnership to provide significant financial support for the global response to HIV/AIDS, TB, and malaria. The United States contributes more to the Global Fund than any other donor. By the end of 2009, the Global Fund had committed to provide $5.3 billion toward malaria proposals in 83 countries.[7]
- **The World Bank:** In 2005, the World Bank launched the World Bank Booster Program for Malaria Control in Africa. The Booster Program is implemented in 18 countries and supports the rapid scale-up of preexisting malaria control interventions and works to strengthen in-country procurement and supply-chain capacity, monitoring and evaluation, and health planning. Funding by the World Bank on malaria control has increased eightfold since 2005.
- **World Health Organization:** WHO is the authority for health within the United Nations system. It is responsible for shaping the global

health research agenda, setting norms and standards, articulating evidence-based policy options, providing technical support to countries, and monitoring global health trends. WHO's Global Malaria Program (GMP) promotes global malaria policies and intervention guidelines, provides technical assistance to malaria programs, and supports research and development of anti-malarial drugs and insecticides.

- **Roll Back Malaria (RBM) Partnership:** The RBM Partnership was created in 1998 by WHO, United Nations Children's Fund (UNICEF), United Nations Development Program (UNDP), and the World Bank to facilitate coordination of malaria activities and optimal use of resources. The RBM Partnership has 500 partners, including malaria-endemic countries, Organization for Economic Cooperation and Development (OECD) donor governments, multilateral organizations, the private sector, NGOs, foundations, research institutions, and ex-officio members. The Coordinator of PMI currently sits on the RBM Partnership Board.
- **United Nations Children's Fund (UNICEF):** UNICEF supports malaria programs through its work on child survival and development. UNICEF assists in developing national malaria plans and policies; monitoring and evaluation; and supplying, procuring, and distributing malaria commodities. According to UNICEF, it is the world's largest procurer and deliverer of ITNs.[8] UNICEF and USAID have a "Malaria Control Partnership" to support malaria programming and commodity procurement, supply, and distribution.
- **American Red Cross:** The American Red Cross malaria programs support distribution of ITNs, community education on the threat of malaria and the proper use of ITNs, and operational research on the effectiveness of ITNs.
- **Bill and Melinda Gates Foundation:** The Gates Foundation advocates increased support for malaria and funds the development of new tools to treat, diagnose, and prevent malaria. The foundation hopes to have supported the development of a malaria vaccine by 2025.[9]

KEY ISSUES IN GLOBAL MALARIA

The 112th Congress will likely be faced with a number of issues regarding the U.S. response to global malaria, including how much assistance to provide and how to best apportion global malaria funds. As Congress debates the role of the U.S. in global malaria control, it might consider the following issues:

- **Insecticide and drug resistance:** Growing instances of drug-resistant malaria and insecticide-resistant mosquitoes threaten global malaria control, particularly in Africa. There are currently no alternatives to available forms of insecticides and treatments. Some health experts argue that anti-malaria resources should prioritize drug and insecticide resistance, including efforts to improve drug quality control, resistance monitoring and surveillance, and research and development of new forms of malaria drugs.
- **Health System Strengthening:** Weak health systems have been a major impediment to successful malaria prevention and treatment. In particular, shortages in health care personnel and weak supply chain networks have limited the delivery of essential commodities for malaria control. There is some disagreement within the global health community about whether PMI has had a beneficial or detrimental impact on the broader functioning of health systems.
- **Control vs. elimination:** There is debate within the global health community over the degree to which the international community should commit itself to malaria control (reducing the disease burden to a level at which it is no longer a public health problem) or malaria elimination (reducing incidence of infection to zero in a defined geographic). While the majority of international funding for malaria efforts in the past decade have been focused on control efforts, a number of experts have argued that efforts should increasingly focus on elimination of the disease. Key issues affecting the debate over control versus elimination include whether countries have the capacity to support more ambitious programs, whether donor assistance is predictable enough to support elimination efforts, and how the international community can avoid any potentially detrimental consequences of an elimination campaign, such as increased insecticide and drug resistance.

End Notes

[1] All data in this section is from World Health Organization (WHO), Global Malaria Program, *World Malaria Report*, 2010, http://whqlibdoc.who.int/publications/2010/9789241564106_eng.pdf.

[2] All data in this section is from WHO, Global Malaria Program, *World Malaria Report*, 2010.

[3] For an explanation of the countries included in each WHO Region, see "WHO Regional Offices," http://www.who.int/about/regions/en/index.html.

[4] USAID, HHS, CDC, and Department of State, *Lantos-Hyde United States Government Malaria Strategy: 2009-2014*, April 25, 2010, http://www.fightingmalaria.gov/resources

[5] WHO, *World Malaria Report*, 2009, p. 57, *http://whqlibdoc. who. int/publications/ 2009/9789241563901_eng.pdf.*

[6] Global Fund to Fight for AIDS, Tuberculosis, and Malaria, *Global Fund 2010 Innovation and Impact*, Progress Report 2010, p. 4.

[7] Ibid.

[8] UNICEF website, "UNICEF in Action: Malaria," http://www.unicef.org/health

[9] Bill and Melinda Gates Foundation website, "Malaria: Our Approach," *http://www. gatesfoundation.org/topics/Pages/* malaria.aspx#.

In: Global Malaria Threat and the U.S. Response ISBN: 978-1-61324-572-9
Editor: Robert N. Moynihan

Chapter 2

LANTOS-HYDE UNITED STATES GOVERNMENT MALARIA STRATEGY 2009–2014

USAID

EXECUTIVE SUMMARY

Malaria prevention and control is a major U.S. foreign assistance objective and is a core component of a comprehensive U.S. Government (USG) Global Health Initiative (GHI), announced in May 2009 by President Barack Obama to reduce the burden of disease and strengthen communities around the world. The 2008 Tom Lantos and Henry J. Hyde Global Leadership against HIV/AIDS, Tuberculosis, and Malaria Act (Lantos/Hyde Act) authorizes up to $5 billion in USG funding for malaria prevention and control for the period FY2009–2013. This Act calls for the development of a comprehensive, multiyear USG strategy to combat malaria globally and strengthen the capacity of the United States to be an effective leader of international efforts to reduce the burden of malaria.

For the purposes of planning, the proposed Lantos-Hyde United States Government Malaria Strategy (USG Malaria Strategy) reflects a six-year horizon (2009–20 14) consistent with the duration of the Global Health Initiative. An evaluation of the activities under the USG Malaria Strategy will take place in the latter half of 2015 to assess progress on activities undertaken through 2014.

The Strategic Vision is that the United States will continue to provide global leadership in reducing preventable malaria deaths to near zero by 2015 and strive toward the ultimate goal of eradication.

As part of the GHI, the USG Malaria Strategy for 2009–2014 proposes an expanded approach to USG-supported malaria control efforts directed at:

- **Achieving Africa-wide impact**, by halving the burden of malaria (morbidity and mortality) in 70 percent of at- risk populations in sub-Saharan Africa (approximately 450 million people), thereby removing malaria as a major public health problem and promoting economic growth and development throughout the region;
- **Limiting the spread of antimalarial multi-drug resistance** in Southeast Asia and the Americas;
- Increasing emphasis on **strategic integration** of malaria prevention and treatment activities with maternal and child health, HIV/AIDS, neglected tropical diseases, and tuberculosis programs, and on **multilateral collaboration** to achieve internationally-accepted goals;
- Intensifying present efforts to **strengthen health systems** and strengthen the capacity of host-country workforces to ensure sustainability;
- Assisting host countries to revise and update their National Malaria Control Strategies and Plans to reflect the declining burden of malaria, and **linking programming of USG malaria control resources to those host- country strategies**; and
- Ensuring a **woman-centered approach** for malaria prevention and treatment activities at both the community and health facility levels, since women are the primary caretakers of young children in most families and are in the best position to help promote healthy behaviors related to malaria.

This USG Malaria Strategy for 2009–2014 also includes important elements of operational research in support of malaria prevention and control efforts that complement the malaria research activities funded by the Department of Health and Human Services (HHS) and executed through the HHS's National Institutes of Health and the Centers for Disease Control and Prevention and by the Department of Defense. This Strategy does not deal with the basic and clinical research being conducted by other USG agencies.

Background

Malaria is a preventable and treatable disease. As recently as 2005, it was estimated to cause between 300 and 500 million illnesses and nearly one million deaths each year. More than 90 percent of these illnesses and deaths occurred among children under five years of age in sub-Saharan Africa. In Asia and the Americas, malaria causes many fewer severe illnesses and deaths, but antimalarial drug resistance is a serious and growing problem. Furthermore, evidence suggests that some drug-resistant strains of malaria have been imported to East Africa from Asia.

The landscape of global malaria control has changed dramatically in the last decade. Three major initiatives have been established to control malaria: the U.S. President's Malaria Initiative (PMI); The Global Fund to Fight AIDS, Tuberculosis and Malaria (Global Fund); and the World Bank Malaria Booster Program. The Roll Back Malaria (RBM) Partnership, created in 1998, has helped to coordinate and harmonize partners' efforts, including a striking increase in private-sector contributions.

As a result, funding for global malaria control has increased sharply since 2000, reaching about $1.5 billion in 2007. According to the RBM Global Malaria Action Plan, in the 109 malarious countries or territories where malaria is endemic, the total costs for malaria prevention and treatment activities and program strengthening worldwide are estimated to range from $6 to $7 billion annually for the next 10 years. Africa accounts for about one-half of those costs.

The President's Malaria Initiative (2005–2010): In June 2005, the U.S. Government announced a new five-year, $1.2 billion initiative to rapidly scale up malaria prevention and treatment interventions in 15 high-burden countries in sub- Saharan Africa. The initiative is led by the U.S. Agency for International Development (USAID) and implemented together with HHS 's Centers for Disease Control and Prevention (CDC). The goal of this initiative is to reduce malaria- related mortality by 50 percent across the 15 focus countries through a rapid scale-up of four proven malaria prevention and treatment measures: insecticide-treated mosquito nets (ITNs); indoor residual spraying (IRS) of insecticides; artemisinin-based combination therapy (ACTs); and intermittent preventive treatment of pregnant women (IPTp).

Selection of the 15 focus countries was based on their malaria burden, the presence of technically sound national malaria control policies, willingness to partner with the United States, and a Global Fund malaria grant. The initiative, which began in 2006, was initially expected to cover a population of 170 million but is now covering 270 million residents in the 15 PMI focus countries (see Table 1 below).

Progress to date: As agreed upon when PMI was launched in 2005, and as a member of the RBM Partnership, PMI does not try to attribute increases in coverage of malaria interventions or reductions in malaria morbidity and mortality to PMI-supported efforts alone. Instead, PMI measures progress toward achieving national and international goals and targets that result from the combined efforts of host country governments and other partners involved in malaria control in that country.

Table 1. President's Malaria Initiative Focus Countries.

Fiscal Year (FY)	Budget	Focus Countries
2006	\$30 million[1]	Round 1: Angola, Tanzania, Uganda
2007	\$135 million[2]	Round 2: Malawi, Mozambique, Rwanda, Senegal (in addition to Round 1 countries)
2008	\$300 million[3]	Round 3: Benin, Ethiopia (Oromia Region), Ghana, Kenya, Liberia, Madagascar, Mali, and Zambia (in addition to Round 1 and Round 2 countries)
2009	\$300 million	All 15 PMI focus countries
2010	\$500 million	All 15 PMI focus countries
TOTAL: \$1 .265 billion		

[1] In addition, Angola, Tanzania, and Uganda also used \$4.2 million in FY05 funds for malaria activities.

[2] This total does not include \$25 million of additional FY07 funding, of which \$22 million was used for malaria activities in the 15 PMI focus countries. In addition, Malawi, Mozambique, Rwanda, and Senegal used \$11.9 million in FY06 funds for malaria activities as allocated by the U.S. Global Malaria Coordinator.

[3] Benin, Ethiopia (Oromia Region), Ghana, Kenya, Liberia, Madagascar, Mali, and Zambia also used \$23.6 million of FY06 and \$42.8 million of FY07 funding (of which \$2.8 million was included in the \$25 million additional FY07 funding) as allocated by the U.S. Global Malaria Coordinator.

In collaboration with national malaria control programs and other major donors, major progress has been made in scaling up malaria prevention and treatment measures across the 15 PMI focus countries. Significant reductions in malaria-related morbidity and 20–30 percent reductions in all-cause childhood deaths (to which malaria is a major contributor) are already being reported from six countries: Ghana, Kenya, Rwanda, Senegal, Tanzania, and Zambia. For example, in Rwanda, (where USAID has been providing funding for malaria activities since 2002 and PMI "jump start" funds beginning in FY2006), a 2008 national survey showed that the frequency of malaria parasitemia fell to less than 3 percent and that under-five childhood mortality fell by 32 percent when compared with 2005; during the same time period, the proportion of children sleeping under an ITN has risen nearly four-fold to 57 percent. In Senegal, there has been a 29 percent reduction in under-five mortality over the same time frame, while household ownership of at least one ITN rose from 36 percent to 60 percent. In Zambia, national survey data showed that between 2006 and 2008 there was a 53 percent decline in the frequency of malaria infection and a 68 percent decline in severe anemia in children under five, and between 2001 and 2007, a 29 percent reduction in deaths in children under five. District-level impact has also been reported in several other countries where ITN usage has already reached high levels and/or large-scale IRS is underway.

PRESIDENT'S MALARIA INITIATIVE (2009–2014)

The 2008 Tom Lantos and Henry J. Hyde Global Leadership against HIV/AIDS, Tuberculosis, and Malaria Act (Lantos/Hyde Act) authorizes up to $5 billion in U.S. Government (USG) funding for malaria prevention and control. This Act provides for the continuation of support to the 15 PMI focus countries and an expansion to other endemic countries. The Act also calls for the development of a comprehensive multi-year USG malaria strategy.

In May 2009, President Obama announced the USG Global Health Initiative (GHI), a six-year, $63 billion commitment to global health. It includes $51 billion to build on the progress made in recent years against malaria, HIV/AIDS, and tuberculosis, together with $12 billion for maternal and child health and neglected tropical diseases programs. This new initiative places renewed USG emphasis on health systems strengthening, program integration, and a woman-centered approach to health development.

Guiding Principles

Malaria prevention and control is a major U.S. foreign assistance objective and is a component of a comprehensive USG global health strategy to reduce the burden of disease and strengthen communities around the world. Full funding of the Lantos/Hyde Act will greatly contribute to broader USG health objectives: reducing global under-five mortality, reducing global maternal mortality, strengthening health systems, and promoting economic growth in Africa.

Vision

The United States will provide global leadership in reducing preventable malaria deaths to near zero by 2015 and in striving toward the ultimate long-term goal of eradication.

Building on the progress and experiences of PMI during the past four years, together with the new approach to international health efforts outlined in the USG Global Health Initiative, the USG Malaria Strategy sets out the following goal and objectives for the period 2009–2014:

Goal

Work with partners to halve the burden of malaria (morbidity and mortality) in 70 percent of the at-risk populations of sub-Saharan Africa, thereby removing malaria as a major public health problem and promoting development throughout the African region.

Objectives

- ***In sub-Saharan Africa***, with full funding over the next five years, the USG will work with National Malaria Control Programs (NMCPs) and partners to accomplish the following:
  - *By 2015, achieve a 70 percent reduction in malaria burden (morbidity and mortality) in the original 15 PMI focus countries,* when compared with the PMI baseline established in 2006/2007;

- *Expand malaria control efforts to reach large areas of the Democratic Republic of the Congo (DRC) and Nigeria and up to seven additional high burden countries,* achieving a 50 percent reduction in malaria burden (morbidity and mortality) in at-risk populations when compared with a 2009–2010 baseline (to be established for these countries). Nigeria and DRC are the two highest burden countries in Africa and account for half of all malaria cases on the continent. The selection of the seven additional countries will be based on population, malaria burden, health infrastructure, and availability of other donor funding.

Altogether, the increased funding will allow USG-supported malaria prevention and treatment measures to be expanded to reach approximately 450 million people, or about 70 percent of the at-risk populations of sub-Saharan Africa.

- ***In Southeast Asia and the Americas***, where antimalarial multidrug-resistance is one of the greatest threats to global malaria control, the USG will work with NMCPs and partners to strengthen efforts to contain the spread of multidrug resistant *Plasmodium falciparum* malaria. This will be accomplished by:
  - Supporting well-functioning antimalarial drug resistance surveillance networks in each country in the region;
  - Establishing national systems to monitor the quality of antimalarial drugs as a means of preventing the introduction and dissemination of sub-standard or counterfeit drugs, which contribute to increased drug resistance; and
  - Contributing to a further reduction in the level of transmission of *P. falciparum* malaria and the number of reported cases in the Greater Mekong Region and the Amazon Basin, with a goal of elimination of malaria in these areas by 2020.

Globally, these efforts will:

- Integrate malaria prevention and treatment activities with maternal and child health efforts, and other major health programs, including HIV/AIDS, neglected tropical diseases, and tuberculosis;
- Build the capacity of host-country health systems and workforces, especially related to critical health systems bottlenecks, such as supply chain management, disease surveillance and reporting, monitoring and evaluation, and laboratory diagnostic services;
- Assist countries to revise and update their national malaria control strategies and plans, as appropriate, to reflect the declining burden of malaria, and link programming of USG malaria control resources to those host-country documents; and
- Ensure a women-centered approach to malaria prevention and treatment activities at both the community and health facility levels, since women are the major caretakers of young children who, along with pregnant women, are most vulnerable to the effects of malaria infections.

Funding Availability

The population targeted in Africa will be calibrated to the funding available through the GHI. If less than full funding is appropriated under this program, then the expected reductions in malaria burden, including in children, will be proportionally reduced.

Strategic Principles

The USG Malaria Strategy for 2009–2014 is guided by many of the same general principles in planning, implementing, and evaluating its malaria control activities that were established when PMI was initially launched:

a) Work within existing national malaria control strategies and plans and strengthen the capacity of national institutions and professionals to address the challenges of malaria control and build country ownership and sustainability;

b) Maintain sufficient flexibility and remain responsive to the ever-changing nature of malaria and tailor efforts to the local epidemiologic setting, including efforts to substantially increase the level of integration of malaria activities with maternal and child health, HIV/AIDS, tuberculosis, and neglected tropical diseases;
c) Design and implement activities in a way that will achieve malaria control objectives at the same time that it builds the capacity of host country systems and workforces, while assessing the impact of these efforts on a country-by-country basis;
d) Utilize a woman-centered approach and promote healthy behaviors related to malaria in families;
e) Remain vigilant to emerging threats, such as drug and insecticide resistance, through rigorous monitoring and surveillance;
f) Promote an integrated and sustainable approach to malaria prevention and control, emphasizing the combined use of antimalarial drugs, vector control measures, behavior change interventions, and as they become available, new tools and strategies that have demonstrated efficacy, have been recommended by the World Health Organization (WHO), and have been locally endorsed;
g) Focus interventions on high-risk populations, while scaling up to universal coverage;
h) Coordinate closely with other multilateral and bilateral institutions and donors and their associated working groups and task forces within the broader RBM Partnership, such as the Global Fund, World Bank, WHO, and UNICEF, to ensure that investments are complementary;
i) Expand and leverage public-private partnerships;
j) Coordinate monitoring and evaluation activities with NMCPs and other partners to track progress toward targets using internationally-accepted indicators and to provide data for timely decision-making; and
k) Conduct operational research that helps overcome implementation bottlenecks, contributes to the scale-up of malaria control activities, and identifies the most cost-effective mix of currently recommended interventions under different malaria transmission settings.

Strategy for Sub-Saharan Africa

To achieve its goal of reduction in malaria-related deaths in Africa, the USG Malaria Strategy will continue to focus on countrywide scale-up of a combination of four proven and highly effective interventions in each of the target countries:

- Long lasting insecticide-treated nets (LLINs);
- Indoor residual spraying (IRS) with insecticides;
- Intermittent preventive treatment of pregnant women (IPTp), where appropriate; and
- Treatment with artemisinin-based combination therapies (ACTs), ideally based on a laboratory diagnosis of malaria.

Insecticide-treated nets: The USG supports the RBM framework for LLIN distribution. This is a multipronged approach to scale up ownership and usage of nets through free distribution during national or sub-national campaigns, free or highly subsidized distribution through antenatal and child health clinics, together with strengthening capacity of the private sector to provide subsidized and unsubsidized LLINs at the lowest possible market price. This approach is intended to produce a rapid scale-up of net coverage, ensuring equity for poor, hardto-reach, and vulnerable populations at the same time that it promotes sustainability. In line with goals set forth by RBM, the USG will support universal coverage with LLINs where this is national policy.

Indoor residual spraying: Between 2005 and 2009, PMI supported the introduction or extension of IRS in all 15 PMI focus countries. PMI-funded IRS activities focused on areas with seasonal transmission (where transmission is limited to certain months of the year and is absent or falls to very low levels during other months). This provides year-round protection with a single round of spraying, rather than focusing on areas with year-round transmission where two or more rounds of spraying are required for full protection. Only WHO-approved insecticides will be procured and used for USG-supported spraying programs. To mitigate the spread of insecticide resistance, USG vector control efforts will support a regular rotation of insecticides from different classes. In addition, all USG- supported IRS will continue to follow required environmental assessment procedures as described in the Code of Federal Regulations, Part 216 (22 CFR 216).

Malaria in pregnant women: The USG supports implementation of the WHO-RBM "Strategic Framework for Malaria Control during Pregnancy in Africa." This recommends a three-pronged approach to reduce the burden of malaria infection among pregnant women in areas with moderate to high-level transmission in the African Region: (1) IPTp, which involves the administration of a full, curative treatment with sulfadoxine-pyrimethamine (SP), an antimalarial drug, at pre-defined intervals during pregnancy; (2) ITNs; and (3) effective treatment of malarial illnesses among pregnant women. Since more than 70 percent of pregnant women in Africa attend antenatal clinics at least once during their pregnancy, the provision of IPTp and ITNs during these clinic visits is both feasible and attractive.

HIV infection diminishes a pregnant woman's ability to control *P. falciparum* infections. Consequently, the USG strongly supports efforts to improve diagnosis and prompt and effective treatment as well as prevention of malaria infections during pregnancy as part of a comprehensive package of HIV/AIDS care. This will be done in coordination with the U.S. President's Emergency Plan for AIDS Relief (PEPFAR) in those countries where both programs are working.

Effective diagnosis and treatment of malaria: Timely and accurate diagnosis of malaria is key to the effective management of malaria infections and the prevention of severe malaria and malaria-related deaths. With the spread of antimalarial drug resistance and adoption of newer and more expensive combination therapies, accurate diagnosis has become even more important as a means of targeting malaria therapy and reducing reliance on presumptive treatment of all febrile patients with antimalarial drugs.

The USG Malaria Strategy will continue to support the WHO recommendation that countries experiencing resistance to their current antimalarial drug monotherapies adopt ACTs as first-line treatment for uncomplicated malaria. The USG will provide technical assistance to ministries of health and NMCPs to ensure smooth and effective implementation of newly adopted ACT treatment policies. This includes assistance on forecasting, procurement, testing and monitoring the quality of antimalarial drugs, regulatory response to substandard drugs, distribution, storage and inventory management, and post-marketing surveillance. Since 50 percent or more of all patients with suspected malaria in Africa seek treatment outside the formal health care system, the USG will also support efforts to understand the role of the private sector in malaria treatment and improve provision of appropriate and safe antimalarial drug regimens through private sources. In addition, the USG will support regular monitoring of antimalarial drug resistance to ensure early detection of reduced sensitivity of malaria parasites to artemisinin drugs and the ACTs.

New tools: A number of new malaria control tools are under development. One of these, intermittent preventive treatment in infants (IPTi), has received recent provisional approval from WHO. This strategy involves the administration of an antimalarial drug (usually SP) three times during infancy at the time of routine vaccinations. The strategy will be limited to countries with continuing moderate or high malaria transmission and moderate or lower levels of SP resistance. Once the strategy receives formal approval from WHO, the possibility of IPTi scaleup in countries will be considered.

Although individual control measures may have a significant impact on malaria illnesses and deaths in the short term, lasting and sustainable reductions in malaria burden will depend on an integrated approach using a combination of the above prevention and treatment measures and strengthening health systems and building capacity for local ownership.

Strategy for Southeast Asia and South America

Levels of malaria transmission in Southeast Asia and South America are much lower than in sub-Saharan Africa. Although malaria is responsible for considerable illnesses in these regions, deaths due to malaria are much less common. Because of the lower levels of transmission, immunity to malaria is not acquired during childhood and all age groups and both men and women are at risk of disease. National malaria control programs in these two regions are generally quite strong and are able to meet most of the commodities and services needs for malaria prevention and control.

The spread and intensification of antimalarial drug resistance represents the single most serious challenge to malaria control in Asia and the Americas. In the Mekong Region of Southeast Asia, strains of *P. falciparum* have already developed resistance to chloroquine, SP, and mefloquine, and the recent reports of resistance to artemisinin are particularly alarming. There is also evidence to suggest that in the past Southeast Asia may have been the major source of drug-resistant strains of malaria parasites in East Africa. In the Amazon Basin, high-level resistance to both chloroquine and SP is already present, and there is evidence of early mefloquine resistance, although ACTs remain effective.

The USG has taken a regional approach to supporting malaria control activities in Asia and the Americas, although it also supports activities at the country level. During the last ten years, USAID in collaboration with CDC assisted NMCPs in strengthening antimalarial drug resistance surveillance and updating and implementing national malaria treatment policies based on ACTs, as recommended by WHO. All eight of the countries making up the Amazon Basin of South America and five of the six countries in the Mekong Region of Southeast Asia have now adopted ACTs as their first-line drugs for the treatment of *falciparum* malaria.

The challenge now is to sustain routine monitoring of antimalarial drug resistance to detect early any loss in efficacy of the first- and second-line drugs. With the spread of drug resistance, accurate laboratory-based diagnosis with microscopy or rapid diagnostic tests has become even more important as a means of targeting malaria therapy. Counterfeit or substandard antimalarial drugs are being encountered with increasing frequency as drug resistance drives the cost of malaria treatments higher. This problem is particularly serious in Southeast Asia, where extremely sophisticated counterfeits of several artemisinin drugs and ACTs have been detected. Through its implementing partners, the USG Malaria Strategy will continue to work with the WHO, the U.S. Food and Drug Administration (FDA), host country governments and other U.S. and international groups to ensure the quality of drugs purchased from recommended manufacturers and to establish or strengthen national capabilities for antimalarial drug quality testing.

Given the relatively low levels of malaria transmission in Southeast Asia and South America, when compared with sub- Saharan Africa, targeted efforts in these areas can reduce the spread of antimalarial drug resistance and may ultimately lead to national and/or regional elimination of malaria. For this reason, the USG will support focused activities, such as active case detection and treatment, as well as outreach to hard-to-access groups to reduce further the risk of malaria transmission in the Mekong Region and Amazon Basin.

The USG Malaria Strategy's Long-Term Vision (2015–2040)

The USG Malaria Strategy for 2009–2014 will directly contribute to the RBM Partnership's Global Malaria Action Plan, which aims to achieve and sustain reductions in worldwide malaria deaths and illnesses over the next 10 to 15 years. The long-term goal is the eventual global eradication of the disease by 2040–2050, when the development of new tools such as a malaria vaccine, make that feasible. To reach this goal, the interim targets of the Global Malaria Action Plan are to:

- Achieve universal coverage of at-risk populations with a package of malaria prevention and treatment measures by December 2010 and sustain those interventions until country-level evidence suggests that coverage can be gradually reduced without risking a resurgence of disease;
- Reduce the worldwide number of malaria cases by 50 percent in 2010 and by 75 percent in 2015 when compared with 2000 levels;
- Reduce worldwide malaria deaths from 2000 levels by 50 percent in 2010 and to near zero by 2015; and
- Support progressive elimination of malaria in additional countries from 2015 through 2030.

The USG Malaria Strategy's long-term vision is to build on the lessons learned and successes in malaria control over the last five years to support the goals and targets of the Global Malaria Action Plan. In partnership with host countries, other major donors, such as the Global Fund, the World Bank, the private sector, and nongovernmental and community- based organizations, the USG expects to reach the following milestones:

- By 2015, achieve near-universal coverage of populations at risk of malaria in the 15 original PMI countries with highly-effective malaria prevention and treatment measures. This should result in a 70 percent reduction in malaria burden (illnesses and deaths) in those countries, when compared with the PMI baseline established in 2006–2007. At the same time, the USG will expand malaria control efforts to large areas of Nigeria, DRC, which together account for one-half of all malaria in sub-Saharan Africa, and up to seven additional high-burden countries with a goal of a 50 percent reduction in malaria illnesses and deaths when compared to 2009–20 10 baselines;
- Between 2015 and 2020, assist Southern Africa Development Community (SADC) countries to create a malaria- free zone in southern Africa through the elimination of transmission in four of those countries;

- Between 2015 and 2030, sustain control efforts in the USG-supported countries across Africa, contributing to the progressive creation of malaria-free zones in East, West, and Central Africa. Achieving this milestone will depend on the control of malaria in both Nigeria and DRC, since those two countries account for such a large proportion of all malaria cases in Africa and they share borders with many other countries that are much farther along in their malaria control efforts. For example, DRC alone has common borders with five PMI countries, three of which are already showing significant reductions in under-five childhood mortality;
- Continue to support work to contain the spread of multidrug-resistant malaria in the Mekong and Amazon Regions, with the long-term goal of elimination of *falciparum* malaria, the most severe form of the disease, from those areas; and
- Demonstrate country ownership to prevent and control malaria morbidity and mortality through strong NMCPs with predictable funding and the staff and technical capabilities to implement and oversee national malaria control efforts.

Responding to Reductions in the Levels of Malaria Transmission

Significant progress in reducing malaria-related illnesses and deaths is already being seen in a number of the 15 PMI focus countries and additional progress can be expected in the coming years as major increases in coverage of malaria prevention and treatment measures are achieved and sustained. Under the USG Malaria Strategy and in collaboration with other donors and the host countries, reductions in malaria burden will be achieved and sustained through universal coverage of vector control interventions with improved diagnosis and prompt treatment of malaria infections with safe and highly effective ACTs.

As malaria transmission falls, the use of accurate laboratory diagnosis of infections should increase to ensure that antimalarial drugs are appropriately used and resurgences of malaria are promptly detected. The USG will continue its efforts to expand, strengthen, and improve the quality of malaria microscopic diagnosis in health facilities with laboratories and the use of rapid diagnostic tests for malaria in lower-level health facilities, the private sector, and at the community level.

Malaria transmission may fall heterogeneously within a country, leaving pockets with a significant burden while other areas are nearly free of disease; it is essential therefore to have a well-functioning NMCP that is able to adjust quickly and effectively to changing epidemiologic situations. For this reason, the USG Malaria Strategy will continue to invest in strengthening national capacity for malaria control at central, provincial, and peripheral levels. Valuable lessons also can be learned from experiences in other regions of the world, such as Asia and the Americas, where malaria transmission was reduced to very low levels in the 1970s and 1980s.

As malaria transmission declines, changes in approach to malaria prevention and treatment will also be necessary. For example, the role of IPTp may need to be reexamined. Indoor residual spraying will need to be targeted better to areas where transmission persists at moderate to high levels. With scaled-up prevention measures and improved laboratory diagnosis of malaria, the number of malaria treatments can be expected to decline, but the importance of identifying and appropriately treating other causes of fever will increase. While these changes should result in some savings in the cost of malaria control interventions, the costs of detecting and dealing effectively with resurgences of malaria are likely to increase. Assuming that Global Fund support to malaria control efforts continue at the same or increased levels, it should be possible to gradually reduce USG funding to some of the original 15 PMI countries and apply these savings to support increased efforts in newer focus countries.

Malaria Elimination and Eradication

In sub-Saharan Africa, over the near-term, regional or national malaria elimination may only be possible in selected geographic settings such as islands. In the rest of sub-Saharan Africa, the USG remains committed to aggressive malaria control through the rapid scale-up of proven interventions and the development and use of new technologies that will continue to reduce transmission toward an ultimate goal of malaria eradication. These scale-up efforts will directly contribute to decreasing the malaria burden in endemic areas such that countries or regions within countries might enter the pre-elimination phase. Over the six years covered by this Strategy (2009–2014), the focus of the USG Malaria Strategy in sub-Saharan Africa will be to eliminate malaria as a cause of mortality and reduce transmission and malaria-related illnesses to very low levels.

In the Mekong Region and the South America, where transmission levels are already far lower, the USG will support the elimination of *P. falciparum* malaria as part of the effort to contain multidrug resistance. As part of that investment, the USG will remain closely engaged with working groups pursuing malaria elimination. In addition, the USG will contribute to the rigorous evaluation of malaria programs that have achieved near total cessation of malaria transmission, and review the experience with other successful disease elimination and eradication efforts in order to provide lessons learned.

PMI's Role in the Global Health Initiative

The GHI represents a USG-wide commitment to work with host governments and other multilateral partners and donors to improve global health in a holistic and sustainable fashion. The GHI builds upon the successes of PMI, PEPFAR, and USG-supported tuberculosis efforts and will carry those commitments forward to 2014. It will help expand PMI activities to reach approximately 70 percent of the malaria at-risk populations in sub-Saharan Africa by the end of the initiative.

The USG Malaria Strategy and PMI will contribute to the core principles of the GHI in the following ways:

Woman-Centered Programming

As a part of the Global Health Initiative, PMI will work to ensure that women remain at the center of USG- supported malaria prevention and treatment activities during the next six years. Pregnant women, along with children under five are the two groups most vulnerable to the effects of malaria and, consequently are the targets of most malaria prevention measures. In most families, women play the major role in deciding where and when young children will seek treatment for illnesses. Women are also in a position to play a key role in promoting behavior change related to the use of LLINs, malaria therapy, and IRS. The PMI will work with ministries of health to involve their reproductive health and maternal and child health departments in the development of the annual PMI operational plans and promote closer working relationships between NMCPs and these departments on malaria-related activities. The PMI will also explore ways to include malaria-related prevention and treatment messages within basic education programs.

Strategic Integration and Coordination

Maternal and child health services: Under PMI, malaria prevention and control activities have been implemented as part of integrated maternal and child health services and make a significant contribution to strengthening capacity to deliver these services. Insecticide-treated nets are distributed principally through antenatal care and child health clinics or through integrated campaigns that include other interventions, such as vitamin A supplementation or vaccinations. Intermittent preventive treatment of pregnant women (IPTp) is a key element of antenatal care, and antimalarial drugs are provided as part of antenatal and child health services. This approach will continue under the USG Malaria Strategy for 2009–2014. The PMI will work with ministries of health to involve their reproductive health and maternal and child health departments in the development of the annual PMI operational plans and promote closer working relationships between NMCPs and these departments on malaria-related activities. In addition, PMI will support integrated management of childhood illness programs, implementation of community-based treatment of fever in which childhood pneumonia, malaria, and diarrhea are diagnosed and treated by trained community health workers, and Focused Antenatal Care programs, which deal broadly with a comprehensive package of services for pregnant women during antenatal clinic visits.

Coordination of malaria and HIV/AIDS service delivery: PEPFAR and PMI currently have eleven focus countries in common (Angola, Ethiopia, Ghana, Kenya, Malawi, Mozambique, Rwanda, Tanzania, Uganda, and Zambia). With the expansion of malaria control activities to additional countries under the USG Malaria Strategy for 2009–2014, this list will grow. Successful collaborations between PMI and PEPFAR around LLIN distribution campaigns, strengthening laboratory diagnostic services, and large-scale household surveys have already occurred, and opportunities will be sought to expand this collaboration during the next five years. In addition, over the next six years, PMI and PEPFAR will work to achieve the following:

- Increased integration of health system functions, including strengthening of pharmaceutical management systems, health management information systems, and laboratory diagnostic services;
- The delivery, where appropriate and supportive country policies exist, of packages of community-based services that include both management of fever and HIV/AIDS prevention;
- Increased integration of prevention of mother-to-child transmission, antenatal care, and malaria in pregnancy; and
- Increased integration, where appropriate, of behavior change communication activities.

Where applicable and cost-effective, PMI and PEPFAR will also work to integrate health system and service delivery efforts with other disease control programs such as for tuberculosis and neglected tropical diseases.

Coordination and Multilateral Collaboration

Partnerships are at the heart of the USG Malaria Strategy for 2009–2014. Achieving the ambitious targets for coverage of major malaria interventions and reductions in malaria burden proposed above only can be achieved through a coordinated approach with a broad partner base, both at country and international levels. The USG works closely with host country governments and supports their national malaria control strategies and plans. The PMI has been a major partner in the RBM Partnership since it was created in 1998 and has been critical in helping to define and focus Partnership efforts. During the next five years, the USG will:

- Continue to play a key role in RBM Partnership working groups on case management, malaria in pregnancy, vector control, procurement and supply management, monitoring and evaluation, and harmonization between partners;
- Maintain close working relationships with major multilateral partners, such as WHO, UNICEF, the World Bank, and the Global Fund, as well as private sector groups involved in malaria control;
- Fill gaps in life-saving commodities, through mechanisms such as PMI's emergency commodity fund;
- Continue partnering with nongovernmental and faith-based organizations, which often have strong health service delivery

programs at the community level, where the impact of malaria is greatest; and

- Coordinate with the Office of Foreign Disaster Assistance on issues related to malaria in complex emergency situations.

Host-Country Ownership and Partnership

Since PMI was launched in June 2005, lessons learned from PEPFAR have helped guide PMI's approach to ensuring country ownership of malaria control activities. Annual PMI needs assessments and planning visits are carried out with NMCPs and their international and in-country partners. In line with the principles of the "Three Ones," annual PMI Malaria Operational Plans directly support national malaria control strategies, and PMI program objectives and targets are aligned with those of the host country. Additionally, PMI works with NMCPs to develop costed malaria monitoring and evaluation plans to which all partners can contribute. With the reductions in malaria burden in many countries across Africa, PMI will work with NMCPs to revise and update their malaria control plans.

Health Systems Strengthening, Capacity Building, and Sustainability

Given the high burden malaria imposes on overstretched health systems, malaria control provides an important platform on which to base additional efforts to strengthen these systems. Across malaria-endemic countries in Africa, an average of 25–35 percent of all outpatient clinic visits are for clinically diagnosed malaria. In these same countries, between 20–45 percent of all hospital admissions are caused by malaria. Due to late presentation at a health facility, inadequate clinical management, and frequent unavailability of effective drugs, case fatality rates among hospitalized malaria patients range from 15–35 percent among all age groups. Where effective malaria control has been achieved in high-burden areas, this has resulted in fewer outpatient clinic visits and a dramatic reduction in hospitalizations for malaria. This "unburdening" of the health system frees up health care workers and hospital beds, creating opportunities for the health care systems to function more efficiently.

During the past four years, PMI has supported the sustainability of its programs by strengthening health systems and building the capacities of public and private sector health workers and managers. All PMI activities directly support national malaria control strategies and plans and are implemented with national ministries of health. The USG Malaria Strategy for 2009–20 14 will continue this approach, with the long-term goal of ensuring that the gains achieved with USG and other donor support can be sustained. While the focus will remain on malaria, PMI will work to:

- Improve forecasting, procurement, quality control, storage, and distribution of medicines;
- Strengthen disease surveillance and reporting and program monitoring and evaluation within ministries of health;
- Improve service delivery by integrating malaria prevention and treatment activities with other disease control and maternal and child health programs;
- Help build host country managerial and technical capacity related to malaria control;
- Improve the quality of laboratory diagnostic services; and.
- Support capacity development to train malaria leaders.

As part of its investments in health systems strengthening, the USG will track and measure improvements in the functioning of key health systems (e.g., pharmaceutical management systems, health management information systems) at the country level using a competency based index already being employed by PMI.

Improved Monitoring, Metrics, and Evaluation

Careful monitoring and evaluation of malaria control efforts will be critical to continue documenting the progress and success of global malaria control efforts. Coverage of major malaria interventions will be monitored through nationwide household surveys. The impact of USG and partner efforts will be measured by following changes in all-cause mortality in children under five and by following changes in the prevalence of malaria infections and severe anemia, which is closely associated with malaria in young children.

During the next five years, PMI will continue its close coordination with NMCPs and national and international partners. The PMI will work through the RBM Monitoring and Evaluation Reference Group to standardize data collection and reporting using internationally accepted indicators. As part of this effort, PMI will continue to support host country efforts to develop costed national malaria monitoring and evaluation plans, build and strengthen national and provincial/district-level capacity in monitoring and evaluation, including routine data collection systems for health, passive and active malaria surveillance, data analysis, and use of data for decision making. In keeping with the Lantos/Hyde Act, CDC will advise the U.S. Global Malaria Coordinator on monitoring, surveillance, and evaluation activities and be a key implementer of these activities.

To evaluate whether the mortality reduction goals have been achieved, PMI will examine trends in all-cause child mortality, malaria parasitemia, and severe anemia, coverage of malaria control measures (e.g., LLIN, IRS protection) and other factors influencing all-cause child mortality (e.g., vaccination coverage) and malaria- specific mortality (e.g., rainfall). These trends will be used to establish whether mortality has decreased and whether mortality reductions can be attributed to programmatic efforts. Mathematical models will be used to assist in quantification of the reductions in malaria-specific mortality. PMI will not try to attribute increases in coverage of malaria interventions or reductions in malaria morbidity and mortality to USG-supported efforts alone. Instead, PMI will measure progress toward achieving national and international goals and targets that result from the combined efforts of host country governments and other partners involved in malaria control in that country.

As malaria transmission declines, PMI will help build national capacity for malaria surveillance at the health facility level, and using experience gained in Asia and South America, surveillance will be expanded to community health workers. At the same time, district health teams need to have the capability to respond in a timely fashion, so that any resurgences of malaria can be rapidly contained. With the threat of parasite resistance to antimalarial drugs or anopheline mosquito resistance to insecticides, PMI will also assist countries in establishing systems for routine monitoring of antimalarial drug and insecticide resistance.

Coordinating USG Malaria Research Efforts

Research is essential to the development and deployment of malaria control tools throughout the malaria endemic world. The USG has for many years played a leading role in supporting and conducting research to develop and test malaria control interventions, including IRS, LLINs, IPTp and ACTs, as well as research and development of new prevention and treatment tools, such as malaria vaccines and new antimalarial drugs. In the future, it will be critical to maintain the USG's strategic role in both basic and applied research related to malaria control.

The Lantos/Hyde Act directs the U.S. Global Malaria Coordinator to ensure that the operational and implementation research supported by under this Act is complementary to research conducted by the National Institutes of Health. This will be accomplished through regular meetings of representatives of HHS, National Institutes of Health, CDC, Department of Defense, and USAID to coordinate research agendas and activities. The Act also directs CDC to advise the U.S. Global Malaria Coordinator on operations research priorities and to be a key implementer of this research.

Under the Lantos/Hyde Act, the focus of malaria research will be on answering operational questions of importance to the implementation of malaria prevention and treatment activities of the Initiative. Many of these questions are related to the use and cost-effectiveness of malaria control measures individually and in combination and will include efforts to establish the best mix of interventions at differing levels of transmission. Interventions that operate in similar fashions, such as IRS and LLINs, may be synergistic, antagonistic, or duplicative. Other interventions, such as IPTp in pregnant women and antimalarial drug treatment without diagnostic confirmation, may be appropriate in settings of high malaria transmission, but no longer cost-effective when transmission falls to low levels. With reductions in malaria transmission, opportunities will also arise to monitor changes in the economic impact of malaria.

As new or improved malaria interventions are developed, operational research will be required to see how best they can be incorporated into USG malaria activities. Understanding how well and under what conditions these tools work will be critical to guiding cost-effective and technically sound decisions. Currently, malaria control program managers and their donor partners aim for high-level coverage of all interventions, but as these goals are attained, they face decisions about where and when to scale back. Without operational research, there will be little knowledge or experience to guide such decisions. These operational research activities will also provide excellent opportunities for mentoring and building capacity among host country public health workers and scientists.

USAID will continue its support to malaria vaccine development and research through the Malaria Vaccine Initiative and for antimalarial drug discovery and development through Medicines for Malaria Venture.

It is expected that existing NIH, CDC, and Department of Defense efforts to develop and test new malaria prevention and control tools, such as new antimalarial drugs, insecticides, and malaria vaccines, as well as to train qualified malariologists, entomologists, and malaria researchers will be continued under those agencies' intra- and extramural research programs. These efforts will complement the implementation research to be carried out under the Lantos/Hyde Act.

PMI Governance and Management

The 2008 Lantos/Hyde Act establishes "within the United States Agency for International Development a Coordinator of United States Government Activities to Combat Malaria Globally (Malaria Coordinator)." The Malaria Coordinator "shall coordinate the provision of assistance by working with relevant executive branch agencies, including the Department of State (including the Office of the Global AIDS Coordinator), the Department of Health and Human Services, the Department of Defense, and the Office of the United States Trade Representative; and relevant multilateral institutions, including the World Health Organization, the United Nations Children's Fund, the Global Fund, the World Bank, and the Roll Back Malaria Partnership." For each PMI focus country, an interagency country team composed of USAID and CDC staff will develop a detailed one-year implementation plan describing planned activities, expected results and required budget, based on the national malaria control plan and the experience and results of the previous year's activities. The first year's plan will include a five-year strategy.

The USG Malaria Strategy places a premium on tracking how the Initiative's resources are used; transparency in the way priorities are set and decisions made at the country level; involving other stakeholders; and achieving and documenting results. The Program's management plan stresses:

- Early obligation of congressionally-appropriated funds so that nearly 100 percent of funds are obligated within the same fiscal year with approximately 30 percent obligated during the first quarter of that year;

- Close management of financial pipelines and routine tracking and review of all activities;
- Minimizing lead times for procurement of critical commodities and services;
- Flexibility in working with other donors to fill gaps in core malaria commodities and services, such as funding the distribution of LLINs procured by other partners;
- Maintaining a central emergency procurement fund to help ensure that no country experiences a stock-out of essential commodities each year; and
- Tracking progress toward the Initiative's goals and objectives.

ACCOUNTABILITY

The PMI has placed a high priority on accountability and transparency. All annual country-level malaria operational plans, the USG Malaria Strategy for 2009–2014, and malaria programmatic and technical guidance documents are posted on the Initiative's website (http://www.pmi.gov), once they are approved by the U.S. Global Malaria Coordinator. In addition, all major contracts and agreements related to malaria activities are posted on the web.

In: Global Malaria Threat and the U.S. Response ISBN: 978-1-61324-572-9
Editor: Robert N. Moynihan

Chapter 3

SUSTAINING MOMENTUM AGAINST MALARIA: SAVING LIVES IN AFRICA

USAID

ABBREVIATIONS AND ACRONYMS

ACT	Artemisinin-based combination therapy
AL	Artemether-lumefantrine
BCC	Behavior change communication
CDC	Centers for Disease Control and Prevention
CHW	Community health worker
FANC	Focused antenatal care
FBO	Faith-based organization
FY	Fiscal year
Global Fund	The Global Fund to Fight AIDS, Tuberculosis and Malaria
HHS	Department of Health and Human Services
HIV/AIDS	Human Immunodeficiency Virus/Acquired Immune Deficiency Syndrome
IPTp	Intermittent preventive treatment for pregnant women
IRS	Indoor residual spraying
ITN	Insecticide-treated mosquito net
M&E	Monitoring and evaluation
MCP	Malaria Communities Program
MIP	Malaria in pregnancy

MOH	Ministry of health
N GO	Nongovernmental organization
NMCP	National malaria control program
PEPFAR	U.S. President's Emergency Plan for AIDS Relief
PMI	President's Malaria Initiative
PMTCT	Prevention of mother-to-child transmission of HIV
RBM	Roll Back Malaria
RDT	Rapid diagnostic test
SP	Sulfadoxine-pyrimethamine
UNICEF	United Nations Children's Fund
USAID	U.S. Agency for International Development
USG	U.S. Government
WHO	World Health Organization

"In Africa, where the disease burden is the greatest, many countries are making dramatic gains in reducing theterrible burden of malaria, particularly for the benefit of those most vulnerable, so that malaria is no longer anintractable fact of life. Today, I recommit to work with our partners in this fight."

– U.S. President Barack Obama, World Malaria Day celebration, April 24, 2009

EXECUTIVE SUMMARY

A Dramatic Scale-Up of Malaria Control Interventions

This report outlines the U.S. Government's (USG's) contributions to a dramatic scale-up of malaria prevention and treatment measuresacross 15 President's Malaria Initiative (PMI)-supported countries over the past four years. Many of these countries have reportedsignificant reductions in under-five mortality, and there is strong and growing evidence that malaria prevention and treatment effortsare a major factor in these reductions. Throughout this report, we highlight the USG's role in the scale-up of malaria interventions,training of health workers, support for services and commodities, and health systems strengthening. Progress in malaria control is aresult of the collective actions of African governments; international donors, including the USG, The Global Fund to Fight AIDS,Tuberculosis and Malaria (Global Fund), and World Bank; and nongovernmental organizations.

PMI PROGRESS AT A GLANCE[1]					
	Year1(2006)	Year2(2007)	Year3(2008)	Year4(2009)	Cumulative
Number of people protected by indoor residual spraying	2,097,056	18,827,709	25,157,408	26,965,164	N/A[2]
Number of ITNs procured	1,047,393	5,210,432	6,481,827	15,090,302	27,829,954 (19,301,794 distributed)
Number of ITNs procured byother partners and distributedby PMI	-	369,900	1,287,624	2,966,011	4,623,535
Number of ACT treatments procured	1,229,550	11,537,433	15,454,709	29,616,342	57,838,034 (40,113,517 distributed)[3]
Number of ACT treatments procured by other partners and distributed by PMI	-	8,709,140	112,330	8,855,401	17,676,871
Number of health workerstrained in use of ACTs	8,344	20,864	35,397	41,273	N/A[4]
Number of rapid diagnostictests procured	1,004,875	2,082,600	2,110,000	6,153,350	11,350,825(8,239,825 distributed)[3]
Number of health workerstrained in malaria diagnosis(RDTs and/or microscopy)	-	1,370	1,663	2,856	N/A[4]
Number of IPTp treatments procured	-	1,349,999	1,018,333	1,657,998	4,026,330(3,524,122 distributed)[3]
Number of health workerstrained in IPTp	1,994	3,153	12,557	14,015	N/A[4]

[1] The numbers reported in this table are up-to-date as of January 1, 2010, and include all 15 PMI focus countries. In addition, during 2009, the USG provided support for malaria prevention and control activities in the Democratic Republic of the Congo, Nigeria, and Sudan. As a result, (1) more than 852,000 ITNswere procured and distributed; (2) more than 700 health workers were trained in IPTp, **(Continued)**

and 430,000 IPTp treatments were procured and distributed; and (3)more than 3,000 health workers were trained in the use of ACTs, and more than 6.2 million ACTs were procured, of which 5.4 million were distributed. TheUSG also provided emergency support for an IRS campaign in Zimbabwe in 2009, which protected 929,600 people.

[2] A cumulative count of people protected by indoor residual spraying is not provided since some areas have been sprayed on more than one occasion.

[3] Distributed to health facilities.

[4] A cumulative count of individual health workers trained is not provided since some health workers have been trained on more than one occasion.

Malaria remains one of the major public health problems on the African continent. It is estimated to cause between 300 and 500 million cases and about 900,000 deaths each year, with 90 percent of those deaths in African children under five years of age. Malaria also places a tremendous burden on national health systems and individual families. Economists estimate that malaria accounts for approximately 40 percent of public health expenditures in Africa and causes an annual loss of $12 billion, or 1.3 percent of the continent's gross domestic product. Malaria and poverty are closely linked, and the greatest burden of malaria usually falls on residents of rural areas, where access to health care is most limited.

Launched in 2005, the President's Malaria Initiative (PMI) is a five-year, $1.2 billion expansion of USG resources to reduce the intolerable burden of malaria and help relieve poverty on the African continent. The goal of PMI is to reduce malaria-related deaths by 50 percent in 15 countries with a high burden of malaria (see map on page 10) by expanding coverage of four highly effec-tive malaria prevention and treatment measures to the most vulnerable populations – pregnant women and children under five years of age.

The 2008 Lantos-Hyde Act authorized an expanded PMI program for 2009–20 13. PMI is a key component of the U.S. Government's Global Health Initiative, which was announced by President Obama in May 2009 (see box on page 7). As a result, the PMI strategy was revised to achieve Africa-wide impact by halving the burden of malaria in 70 percent of at-risk populations in sub-Saharan Africa, or approximately 450 million people.

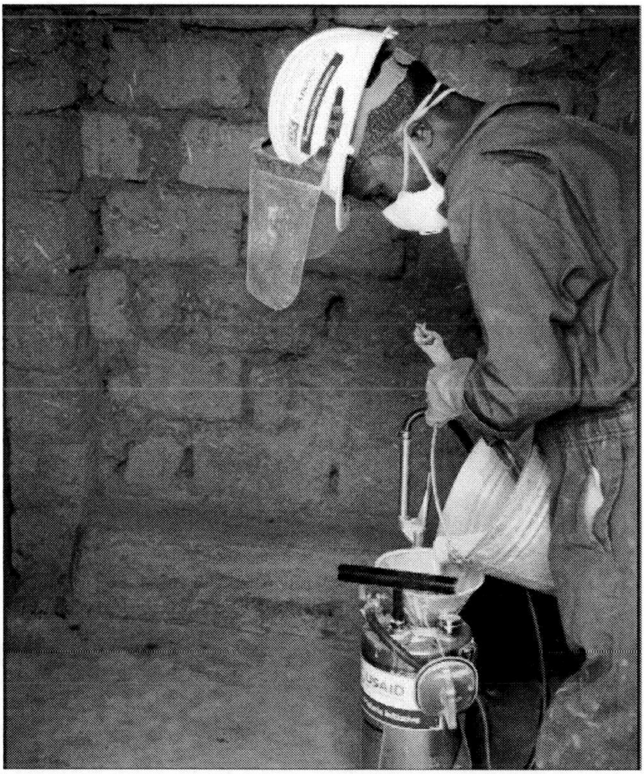

Wearing personal protective equipment, a spray operator prepares his pump during an IRS campaign in Ethiopia. In 2009, PMIsupported IRS activities protected nearly 27 million people.

Scaling Up Coverage of Malaria Interventions

PMI supports four proven and cost-effective prevention and treatment interventions: insecticide-treated mosquito nets (ITNs), indoor residual spraying (IRS) with insecti-cides, intermittent preventive treatment for pregnant women (IPTp), and prompt use of artemisinin-based combination therapies (ACTs) for those who have been diagnosed with malaria. PMI helps countries to scale up access to these interventions nationwide.

Since 2006, substantial progress has been made in scaling up training, focus country capacity building, and malaria prevention and treatment measures across the 15 PMI focus countries, in collaboration with national malaria control programs (NMCPs) and other donors. In 2009 alone, PMI procured more than 15 million long-lasting ITNs, protected approximately 27 million residents by spraying their houses with residual insecticides, and procured more than 29 million ACT treatments (see PMI Progress Table on page 2). The effective and growing collaboration with other donors is evidenced by the nearly 3 million long-lasting ITNs and the 8.8 million ACT treatments procured by other partners, which PMI helped to distribute. In addition, in 2009, PMI trained tens of thousands of people in key aspects of malaria control, including more than 41,000 health workers in the use of ACTs. In all 15 focus countries, PMI provided support to improve the pharmaceutical management of antimalarial drugs and other essential medical products.

Now, four years into PMI, dramatic increases in the coverage of malaria control measures are being documented in nationwide household surveys as a result of the contributions of PMI, prior USG assistance, national governments, and other donors. Nationwide household surveys are the best way to measure population coverage with health interventions; however, because of their cost and effort required, they are only repeated every two to three years in most countries. During the past three years, six PMI countries – Ghana, Kenya, Rwanda, Senegal, Tanzania, and Zambia – reported the results of nationwide household surveys that allow a comparison with earlier nationwide household surveys, which are used as the PMI baseline. In these six countries, household ownership of one or more ITNs increased from the baseline range of 15 to 38 percent to a 2007–2009 range of 33 to 60 percent (see page 13). At the same time, usage of an ITN the night before the survey almost doubled from an average of 22 to 41 percent for children under five and about the same amount for pregnant women. This increased ITN ownership and use, together with an average of 22 million residents protected each year for the past 3 years across the 15 PMI countries by PMIsupported IRS, means that a large proportion of the at-risk populations in these 15 countries are now benefiting from one or more highly effective malaria prevention measures. Over the same period of time, the proportion of pregnant women who received two or more doses of IPTp for the prevention of malaria has increased from a baseline average of 24 to 37 percent. Follow-up nationwide household surveys for the remaining nine PMI focus countries will be completed between 2010 and 2012 to permit an assessment of progress across all 15 PMI countries.

The scale-up of ACTs in sub-Saharan Africa has been slower than that for ITNs, IRS, and IPTp due to several factors, including that most countries only adopted ACTs as their first-line treatment for malaria in 2003–2004. Prior to that time, the World Health Organization (WHO) was recommending that all children under five with a fever be treated presumptively for malaria. With the increasing use of diagnostic testing for patients with suspected malaria, the ACT coverage indicator (proportion of children under five with a fever in the last two weeks who were treated with an ACT) no longer accurately reflects progress with ACT scale-up. Still, there are other indications that access to ACTs has increased dramatically in the 15 PMI focus countries since 2005–2006. For example, in Angola in 2005, ACTs were only available in public health facilities in about 10 of the country's 164 districts. By 2008, ACTs were being used in public health facilities in all 164 districts. Nationwide surveys carried out in late 2008 and early 2009 in Benin, Madagascar, Uganda, and Zambia by ACT Watch, a Bill and Melinda Gates Foundation-funded project, showed that between 66 percent (Benin) and 86 percent (Madagascar) of public health facilities surveyed in the four countries had the first-line ACT in stock on the day of the survey.

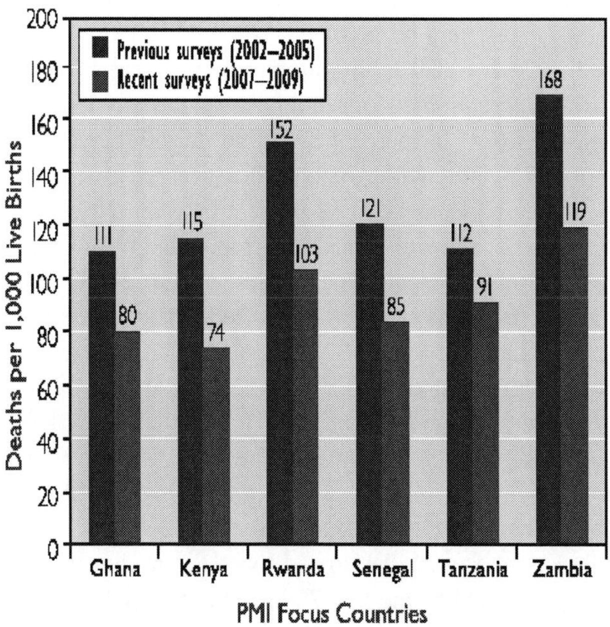

Note: The countries included in this graph are those PMI focus countries for which there are two data points from nationwide household surveys for the indicator.

Figure 1. Reductions in All-Cause Mortality Rates of Children Under Five in Six PMI Countries.

Achieving Impact

In all six PMI countries with paired nationwide house-hold surveys, substantial reductions in all-cause mortality in children under five years of age have been document-ed; these reductions range from 19 to 36 percent (see Figure 1, above). This represents the cumulative effect of malaria funding by PMI, USG prior to PMI, national governments, and other donors.

While a variety of factors may be influencing the decline in under-five mortality rates, there is strong and growing evidence that malaria prevention and treatment efforts are playing a major role in these reductions. For example:

- In **Senegal**, a 30 percent reduction in all-cause mortality in children under five between 2005 and 2008 has been documented. Although several factors may be involved, it is highly likely that this dramatic reduction is due at least in part to rapid increases in the coverage of malaria interventions. Household ownership of one or more ITNs has increased from 36 percent in 2006 to 60 percent in 2008. The proportion of pregnant women who received two or more doses of IPTp increased from 12 to 52 percent between 2005 and 2008. At the end of 2007, Senegal introduced rapid diagnostic tests (RDTs) for malaria in all of its health facilities, and in 2008, 73 percent of all suspected malaria cases were tested. Although no national-level baseline data are available to compare malaria prevalence, fewer than 6 percent of children under five had malaria parasites in the 2008 nationwide survey, a level much lower than would be expected in most West African countries. The U.S. Agency for International Development (USAID) has supported malaria control efforts in Senegal since 1999. In fiscal year (FY) 2006, $2.2 million in PMI funding was provided, followed by $16.7 million in FY 2007, $15.9 million in FY 2008, and $15.7 million in FY 2009.

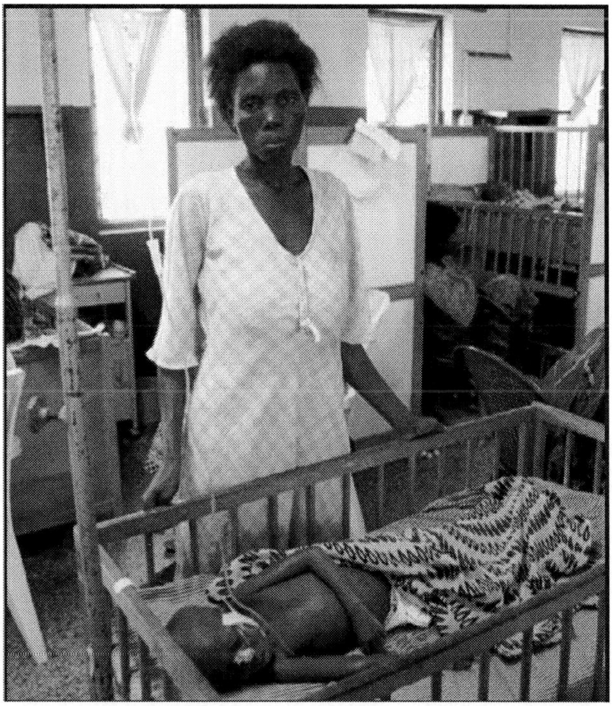

LISA KRAMER/PMI

A mother stands by the crib of her child, who is being treated for severe malaria in Ghana. PMI works with its partners to help ensure that children under five with malaria infections are promptly diagnosed and treated to prevent progression of the infection to a severe, life-threatening illness.

- In **Zambia**, the proportion of households with at least one ITN has increased from 38 percent in 2006 to 62 percent in 2008. More importantly, the use of ITNs by children under five almost doubled from 24 percent in 2006 to 41 percent in 2008. The National Malaria Control Program of Zambia estimates that, since 2003, more than 7 million ITNs have been distributed throughout the country. During the same time period, the prevalence of anemia among children six months to five years of age declined by 71 percent, from 14 to just under- 4 percent, and malaria parasite prevalence dropped from 22 to 10 percent. It is highly likely that these results contributed significantly to the drop in all-cause under- five mortality from 168 deaths per 1,000 live births in 2002 to 119 per 1,000 in 2007. USAID has supported malaria control efforts in Zambia since 2002, including

$7.6 million in FY 2006. PMI provided $9.5 million in FY 2007, followed by $14.9 million in FY 2008, and $14.7 million in FY 2009.

- Analysis of household survey data from **Rwanda** showed that between 2005 and 2008, ITN use in children under five increased from 13 to 58 percent. Over approximately the same time period, the proportion of hospital deaths attributed to malaria fell from 41 to 16 percent. All-cause mortality in children under five also declined by 32 percent between 2005 and 2008. USAID has supported malaria control efforts in Rwanda since 2002. In FY 2006, PMI provided $1.5 million in funding, followed by $20 million in FY 2007, $16.9 million in FY 2008, and $16.3 million in FY 2009.
- In **Tanzania**, all-cause under-five mortality fell from 112 deaths per 1,000 live births in 2005 to 91 per 1,000 in 2007. At about the same time, household ownership of ITNs increased from 23 percent in 2005 to 38 percent in 2007. A recent survey showed that children who slept under an ITN in Tanzania were 40 percent less likely to have malaria parasites in their blood than children who did not sleep under an ITN. In the capital, Dar es Salaam, malaria prevalence fell from 24 percent in 2004 to just 4 percent in 2008, and the prevalence of severe anemia in children six months to five years of age fell by 30 percent between 2004 and 2007. USAID supported malaria control efforts in Tanzania between 1999 and 2005, including $2 million in FY 2005. Beginning in FY 2006, PMI provided $11.5 million in funding, $31 million in FY 2007, $33.7 million in FY 2008, and $35 million in FY 2009.

PMI – A Partner in Malaria Control

PMI is committed to working with a broad range of partners, most importantly national governments and NMCPs, as well as multilateral and bilateral institutions and private sector organizations (see Partners Table on page 6). During the past year, PMI expanded collaboration with the private sector, nongovernmental organizations (NGOs), and faith-based organizations (FBOs). groups often have strong bases of operation in served rural areas, where the burden of malaria is greatest. The Malaria Communities Program (MCP), launched in December 2006, catalyzes partnerships with small national and international NGOs and FBOs.

To date, MCP has awarded 20 grants to 18 organizations That are implementing activities in 12 PMI countries. In total, PMI has supported nearly 200 nonprofit organiza-tions; more than 45 of these are faith based.

Examples of PMI Partners in Malaria Control

Multilateral and Bilateral Partners	Private Sector and Foundations
• Roll Back Malaria Partnership • United Nations Secretary-General's Special Envoy for Malaria • World Health Organization • United Nations Children's Fund (UNICEF) • The Global Fund to Fight AIDS, Tuberculosis and Malaria (Global Fund) • World Bank • United Kingdom Department for International Development	• Malaria No More • Global Business Coalition • Bill and Melinda Gates Foundation • United Nations Foundation • (Nothing but Nets) • ExxonMobil Foundation • Clinton Foundation • Carter Center

The success of PMI is linked to the efforts of other major donors. At the global level, PMI sits on the board of directors of the Roll Back Malaria (RBM) Partnership and is an active member of the U.S. Government's delegation to the Global Fund. At the country level, PMI staff members actively participate in malaria stakeholders groups, including the Global Fund Country Coordinating Mechanism. PMI staff members play an active role in all RBM working groups, including the Monitoring and Evaluation Reference Group. During the past four years, PMI, the ExxonMobil Foundation, Malaria No More, and other donors contributed funding to the Harmonization Working Group of the RBM Partnership to improve the success rate of African countries applying for Global Fund malaria grants. As a result of this support, in Rounds 7 through 9, the success rate of Global Fund malaria proposals from countries that received technical support from the Working Group nearly doubled from the 32 percent rate in Round 6. PMI also works with WHO and other technical partners to reach consensus on issues such as how best to use microscopic diagnosis and RDTs in different epidemiological and clinical settings; how to improve quality standards for antimalarial drugs, especially ACTs; and how to roll out community- based treatment of malaria with ACTs.

Integration with Maternal and Child Health Programs

Malaria prevention and control activities, including those supported by PMI, are a cornerstone of comprehensive maternal and child health services in Africa and make a significant contribution to strengthening capacity to deliver those services. ITNs are distributed principally through antenatal and child health clinics or through integrated campaigns that include other interventions, such as vitamin A supplementation or vaccinations. Evidence suggests that this approach increases the number of women who attend these facilities and campaigns.

IPTp is a key element of antenatal care, and antimalarial drugs are provided as part of antenatal and child health services. PMI also supports integrated management of childhood illness programs; implementation of community-based treatment of fever in which childhood pneumonia, malaria, and diarrhea are diagnosed and treated by trained community health workers; and focused antenatal care programs that provide a comprehensive package of services for pregnant women during antenatal clinic visits.

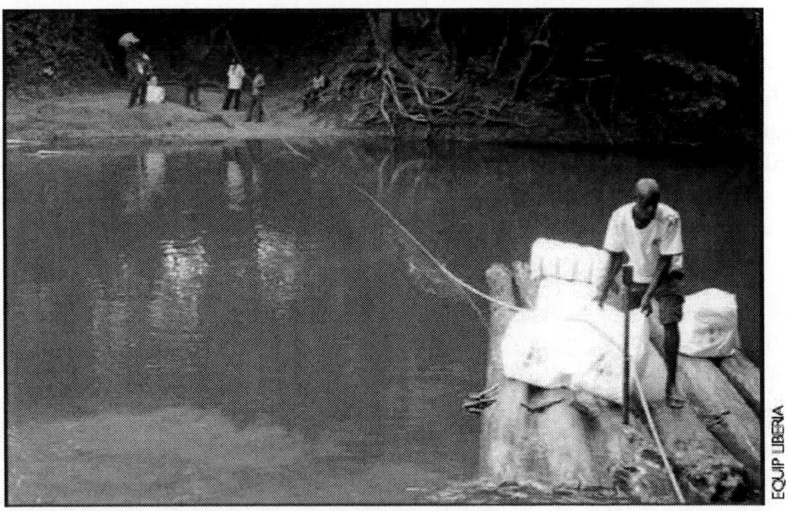

Men ferry bales of ITNs across a river during a net distribution campaign in Nimba County, Liberia, that involved a Malaria Communities Program grantee, Liberian government officials, and PMI implementing partners. More than 180,000 nets were distributed during the campaign.

PMI AND THE GLOBAL HEALTH INITIATIVE

Malaria prevention and control is a major foreign assistance objective of the USG and is a core component of President Barack Obama's Global Health Initiative, a six-year, comprehensive effort announced in May 2009 to reduce the burden of disease and promote healthy communities and families around the world. The U.S. Congress has authorized a substantial increase in resources for malaria prevention and control for the period of FY 2009–2013 and calls for a multi-year USG strategy to combat malaria globally.

As part of the Global Health Initiative, the USG has developed an expanded PMI strategy directed at:

- **Achieving Africa-wide impact** by halving the burden of malaria (morbidity and mortality) in 70 percent of at-risk populations in sub-Saharan Africa (approximately 450 million people), thereby removing malaria as a major public health problem and promoting economic growth and development throughout the region;
- Increasing emphasis on **strategic integration** of malaria prevention and treatment activities with maternal and child health, HIV/AIDS, neglected tropical diseases, and tuberculosis programs, and on **multilateral collaboration** to achieve internationally accepted goals;
- Intensifying current efforts to **strengthen host country health systems** to ensure sustainability;
- Assisting host countries to revise and update their national malaria control strategies and plans to reflect the declining burden of malaria, and linking programming of USG malaria control resources to those host country strategies;
- Ensuring a **women-centered approach** for malaria prevention and treatment activities at both the community and health facility levels, since women are the primary caretakers of young children in most families and are in the best position to help promote healthy behaviors related to malaria; and
- Limiting the threat of malaria multidrug resistance in Southeast Asia and the Americas.

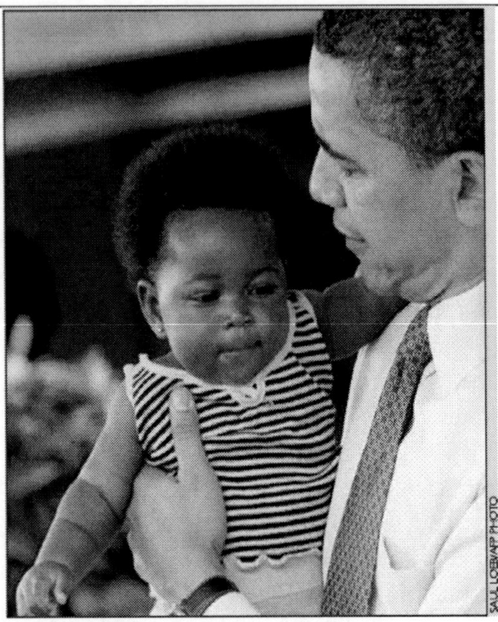

President Barack Obama holds a child during a tour of the La General Hospital in Accra, Ghana, in July 2009. The U.S. Government's commitment to fight malaria is a key component of our nation's foreign assistance strategy and the Global Health Initiative.

Building Capacity of National Health Systems

Both directly and indirectly, PMI resources help build health systems and strengthen overall capacity in host government ministries of health (MOHs) and NMCPs. In highly endemic countries, MOH statistics indicate that malaria often accounts for up to 50 percent of pediatric outpatient visits and hospital admissions. By reducing the burden of malaria in these countries, PMI aims to facilitate the use of critical resources and allow overstretched health workers to concentrate on controlling other childhood illnesses, such as diarrhea and pneumonia. PMI's goal is to enable national governments to be able to control malaria on their own. MOHs and NMCPs must be able to provide leadership combined with technical and managerial skills to plan, implement, evaluate, and adjust, as necessary, their malaria control efforts. Effective NMCPs require staff with expertise in a variety of fields, including entomology, epidemiology, case management, monitoring and evaluation, laboratory diagnosis, supply chain management, behavior change communications, and financial management. In 2009, PMI efforts to strengthen health systems included:

- Providing $9 million in FY 2009 funding for pharmaceutical management activities to help MOHs, NMCPs, and national essential drugs programs improve the forecasting; procurement; quality control; storage; and distribution of antimalarial and other drugs, and for training and supervision of pharmacy and medical store staff and health workers to ensure the correct usage of these drugs;
- Funding for the training of more than 41,000 health workers on case management with ACTs, more than 2,800 in malaria laboratory diagnostics, and morethan 14,000 in IPTp;
- Supporting NMCPs to collect and report data of high quality by conducting routine surveys, strengthening national health management information systems and malaria surveillance programs, and improving epidemic detection and response;
- Providing PMI resident advisors who give direct technical advice and management support to the staff of NMCPs; and
- Collaborating with NMCPs and other partners, such as the U.S. President's Emergency Plan for AIDS Relief (PEPFAR) and WHO, to strengthen laboratory diagnosis of malaria. These efforts to upgrade laboratory services help improve the overall quality of primary health care, diagnosis, and treatment.

Malaria Research

The U.S. Government is committed to significantly reducing the global burden of malaria by supporting research through a coordinated and collaborative approach. The USG malaria research portfolio involves several USG agencies, including the Centers for Disease Control and Prevention (CD C) of the Department of Health and Human Services (HHS), the National

Institutes of Health of the HHS, the Walter Reed Army Institute of Research of the Department of Defense, and USAID. These USG agencies work with a wide range of partners that include other government agencies, private companies, universities, research institutes, and non-governmental organizations. Highlights of advances in USG-supported malaria research include basic malaria biology, vaccine and drug development, and operational research to improve project implementation and impact.

Looking Ahead

An impact on malaria-related illnesses and deaths is already being seen, providing encouragement that malaria can be controlled and removed as the major public health problem on the African continent. In spite of this progress, however, we cannot afford to be complacent. Weak health infrastructures hamper malaria and other disease control programs and threaten the sustainability of these efforts. Together with our partners, PMI is tackling these challenges. With the increased funding for malaria under the Global Health Initiative, the USG has the opportunity to expand malaria prevention and treatment efforts across the continent.

For more information about PMI, please visit http://www.pmi.gov.

PMI FUNDING SUMMARY		
Fiscal Year (FY)	**Budget**	**Focus Countries**
2006	$30 million[1]	Round 1 : Angola, Tanzania, and Uganda
2007	$135 million[2]	Round 2: Malawi, Mozambique, Rwanda, and Senegal (in addition to Round 1 countries)
2008	$300 million[3]	Round 3: Benin, Ethiopia (Oromia Region), Ghana, Kenya, Liberia, Madagascar, Mali, and Zambia (in addition to Round 1 and Round 2 countries)
2009	$300 million	All 15 PMI focus countries
2010	$500 million	All 15 PMI focus countries
TOTAL: $1.265 billion		

[1] In addition, Angola, Tanzania, and Uganda also used $4.2 million in FY 2005 funds for malaria activities.

[2] This total does not include $25 million of additional FY 2007 funding, of which $22 million was used for malaria activities in the 15 PMI focus countries. In addition, Malawi, Mozambique, Rwanda, and Senegal used $11.9 million in FY 2006 funds for malaria activities as allocated by the U.S. Global Malaria Coordinator.

[3] Benin, Ethiopia (Oromia Region), Ghana, Kenya, Liberia, Madagascar, Mali, and Zambia also used $23.6 million of FY 2006 and $42.8 million of FY 2007 funding (of which $2.8 million was included in the $25 million additional FY 2007 funding) as allocated by the U.S. Global Malaria Coordinator.

PMI Background

PMI Structure: PMI is an interagency initiative led by USAID and implemented with CDC. It is overseen by the U.S. Global Malaria Coordinator, who is advised by an Interagency Steering Group made up of representatives of USAID, CDC/HHS, Department of State, Department of Defense, National Security Council, and Office of Management and Budget.

PMI Country Selection: The 15 focus countries were selected and approved by the Coordinator and the Interagency Steering Group using the following criteria:

- High malaria disease burden;
- National malaria control policies consistent with the internationally accepted standards of WHO;
- Capacity to implement such policies;
- Willingness to partner with the United States to fight malaria; and
- Involvement of other international donors and partners in national malaria control efforts.

PMI Approach: PMI is organized around four operational principles based on lessons learned from more than 50 years of USG experience in fighting malaria, and experience gained from implementation of PEPFAR, which began in 2003. The PMI approach involves:

- Use of a comprehensive, integrated package of proven prevention and treatment interventions;
- Strengthening of health systems and integrated maternal and child health services;
- Strengthening of NMCPs and capacity building for country ownership of malaria control efforts; and
- Close coordination with international and in-country partners.

PMI works within the overall strategy and plan of the host country's NMCP, and planning and implementation of PMI activities are coordinated closely with each MOH.

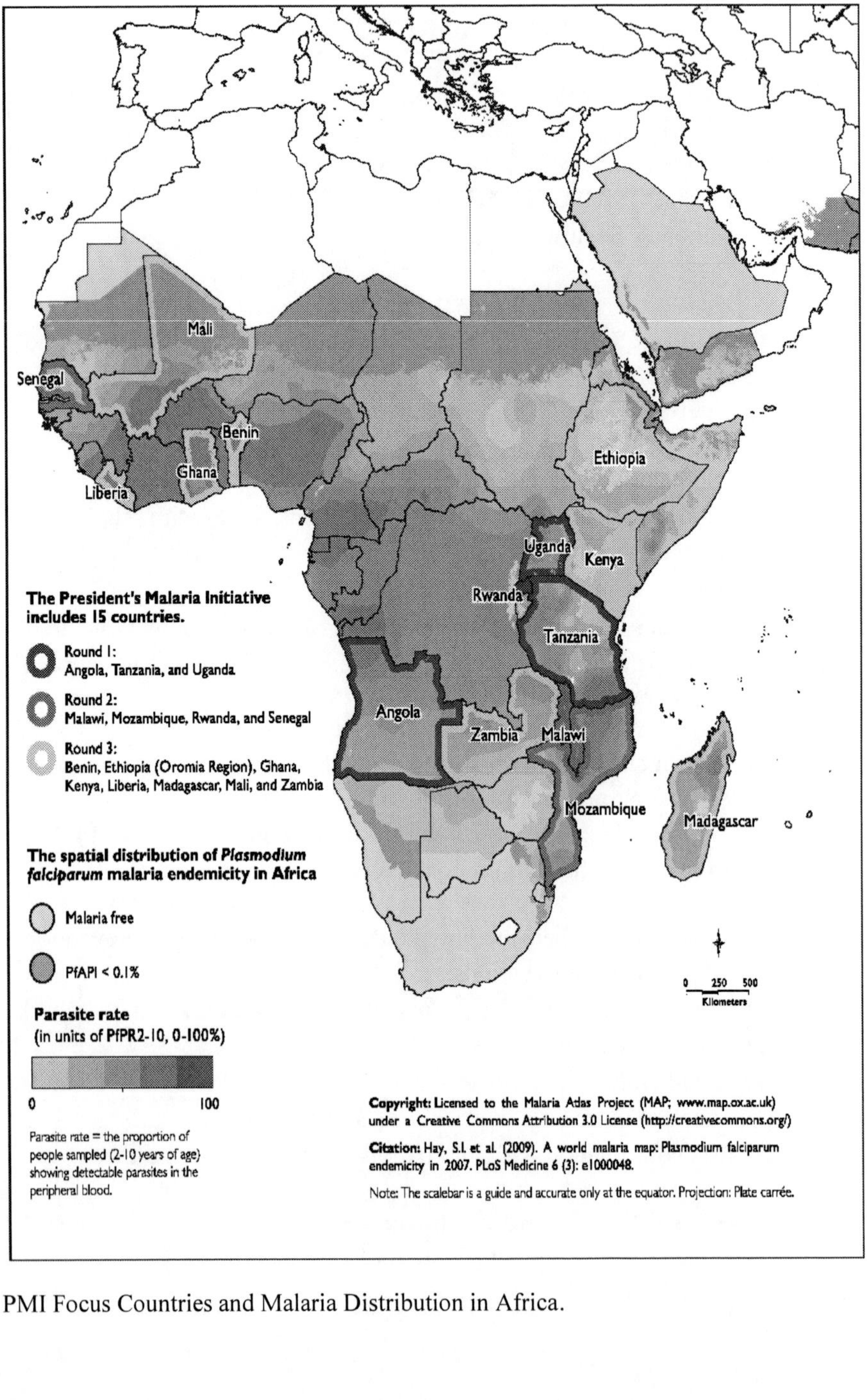

PMI Focus Countries and Malaria Distribution in Africa.

1. Prevention – Insecticide-Treated Mosquito Nets

"As we look ahead, we must embrace core operating principles that worked effectively in the past. In the wakeof the massive effort to scale up to universal coverage of insecticide-treated nets, including in some of the mosthard-to-reach places on the planet, we must continue to sustain high coverage levels."

– Rear Admiral R.T. Ziemer, USN (ret), U.S. Global Malaria Coordinator, October 1, 2009

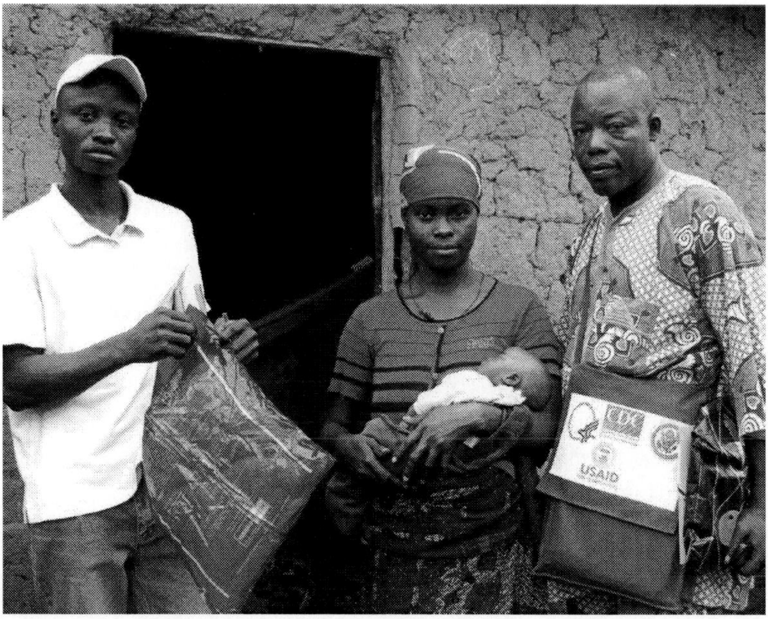

In Benin, Catherine Degboesse and her newborn baby receive a free insecticide-treated mosquito net from Simon Kpossa (left), amember of the Ministry of Health's net distribution team. Across Africa, PMI supports a broad range of strategies to prevent andtreat malaria, targeting vulnerable populations—children under five and pregnant women.

Since malaria in Africa is transmitted by mosquitoes that bite predominantly at night, sleeping under a mosquito net treated with an insecticide that repels mosquitoes and kills those that land on the netting can greatly reduce the risk of infection. Insecticide-treated nets (ITNs) have been shown to reduce all-cause mortality in children under five years of age by about 20 percent and malarial illnesses among children under five and pregnant women by up to 50 percent. The insecticides used to treat the nets have been approved for safety and efficacy by the World Health Organization (WHO). Long-lasting ITNs have the insecticide bound to or incorporated within the netting material during production, enabling the nets to maintain their full protective effect through at least 20 washes or approximately three years of regular use. Long-lasting ITNs have now been adopted by all national malaria control programs (NMCPs) and during the past two years, all PMI procurements and the vast majority of all ITNs procured in Africa since 2005 have been long-lasting ITNs.

Since its launch in 2005, PMI has focused on scaling up ITN coverage in all 15 focus countries. Although ITN activities are tailored to local conditions and capacities within each country, PMI's approach to increasing coverage with ITNs follows certain general principles:

- Targeting the most vulnerable populations – children under five and pregnant women – while working to expand to universal coverage of ITNs for all residents at risk, according to the national strategy;
- Removing cost as a barrier to ITN ownership through provision of free ITNs to the poorest and most vulnerable groups, while allowing market segmentation (offering different styles of ITNs at different prices through a variety of outlets) to help promote markets for and increase access to low-cost or highly subsidized nets for those who can afford them;
- Supporting mass ITN distribution, often integrated with immunization or other health campaigns, to rapidly achieve high ITN coverage;
- Sustaining high ITN coverage through the use of existing platforms for routine net distribution, such as antenatal and child health clinics; and
- Promoting demand for and consistent use of ITNs through behavior change communication (BCC) activities.

PMI ITN Summary

In 2009 alone, PMI procured more than 15 million ITNs. Since it began in 2005, PMI has procured more than 27 million ITNs and has assisted with the distribution of another 4.6 million ITNs procured by other donors. PMI also supported the direct sale of more than 5 million nets and the distribution of nearly 3 million nets that were redeemed at retail outlets through subsidized voucher programs (see table below).

PMI ITN SUMMARY TABLE					
Indicator[1]	**PMI Year 1 (2006)**	**PMI Year 2 (2007)**	**PMI Year 3 (2008)**	**PMI Year 4 (2009)**	**Cumulative**
ITNs procured	1,047,393	5,210,432	6,481,827	15,090,302	27, 829,954 (19,301,794 distributed)
ITNs distributed through voucher programs with PMI support	-	496,607	1,439,706	771,342	2,707,655
ITNs sold with PMI marketing support	586,284	1,702,093	2,407,065	687,404	5,382,846
ITNs procured by other partners and distributed with PMI support	-	369,900	1,287,624	2,966,011	4,623,535

[1] The numbers reported in this table are up-to-date as of January 1, 2010, and include all 15 PMI focus countries. In addition, during 2009, the USG provided support for ITN activities in the Democratic Republic of the Congo, Nigeria, and Sudan; more than 852,000 ITNs were procured and distributed with USG support. For data by country, see Appendix 2.

ITN Coverage Rates

PMI's ITN coverage targets are:

- more than 90 percent of households with a pregnant woman and/or children under five will own at least one ITN;
- 85 percent of children under five will have slept under an ITN the previous night; and
- 85 percent of pregnant women will have slept under an ITN the previous night.

PMI is making progress toward reaching these targets. For example, in **Ghana**, **Rwanda**, **Senegal**, **Tanzania** (both the Mainland and **Zanzibar**), and **Zambia**, significant gains have been made in terms of ITN ownership and use among pregnant women and children under five (see Figures 1–3).

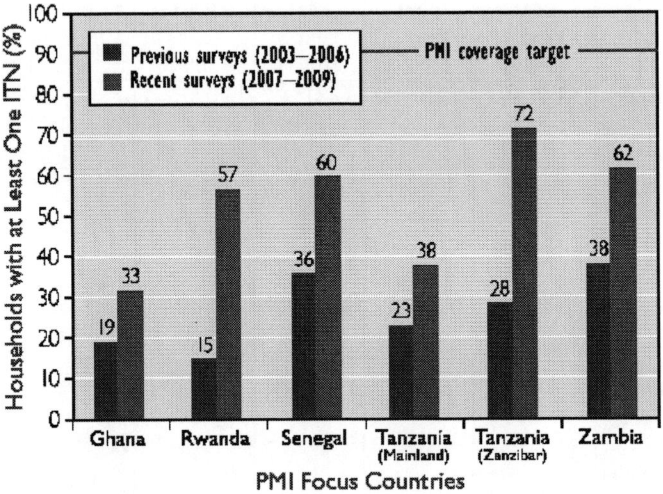

Figure 1. Increases in ITN Ownership in Selected PMI Countries.

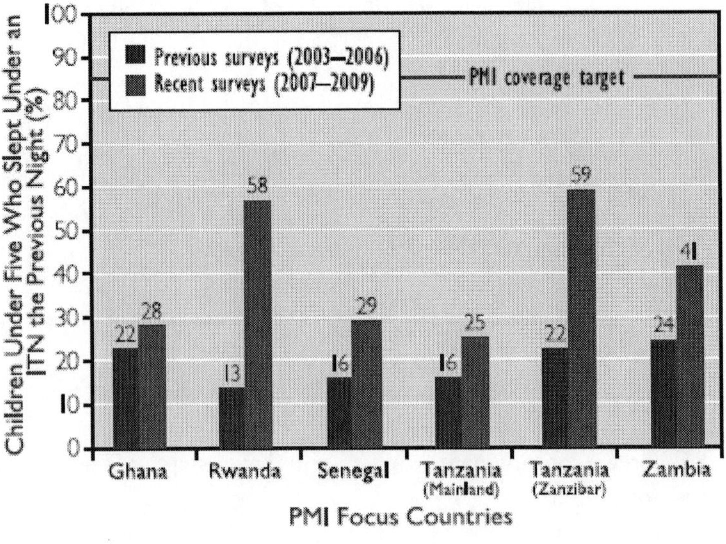

Figure 2. Increases in ITN Use among Children Under Five in Selected PMI Countries.

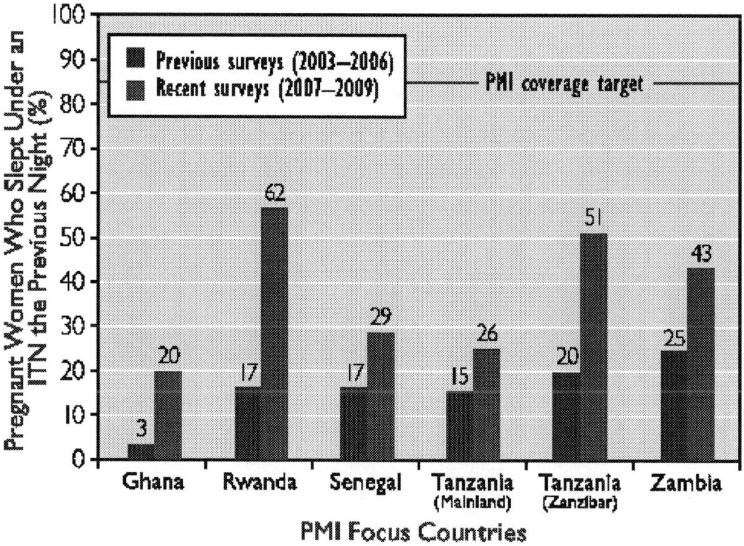

Figure 3. Increases in ITN Use among Pregnant Women in Selected PMI Countries.

Scaling Up Ownership of ITNs through Mass Campaigns

Distribution of free ITNs as part of mass immunization or child health campaigns is an attractive approach to rapidly scale up net ownership, and evidence suggests that receiving a free net may increase attendance of mothers and their children at these campaigns. Universal coverage of the entire population at risk of malaria, along with usage rates above 60 percent among children under five, has been shown to greatly increase the impact of ITNs on malaria morbidity and mortality. Nearly all 15 PMI focus countries have adopted universal coverage as their national strategy.

During the past year, significant progress has been made in scaling up ITN ownership in PMI countries:

- In Senegal, PMI assisted the NMCP with its first nationwide distribution of nearly 2.3 million free ITNs to children under five in June and October 2009. This campaign included vitamin A supplementation and deworming and involved numerous local and international partners. PMI contributed 380,000 ITNs and 30 percent of operational costs, including transport of all nets to 57 health districts and printing and distribution of campaign guides, data collection tools, and BCC materials to promote year-round use of nets. PMI also supported the participation of 1,850 Senegalese Red Cross Society volunteers in the distribution campaign, as well as post-campaign visits to more than 120,000 households to help families hang their nets and to counsel them about malaria. Advocacy by PMI resulted in donations of an additional 86,000 nets from the Canadian Red Cross, the Against Malaria Foundation, and Sumitomo Chemical Company, and in funding for operational costs from World Vision.

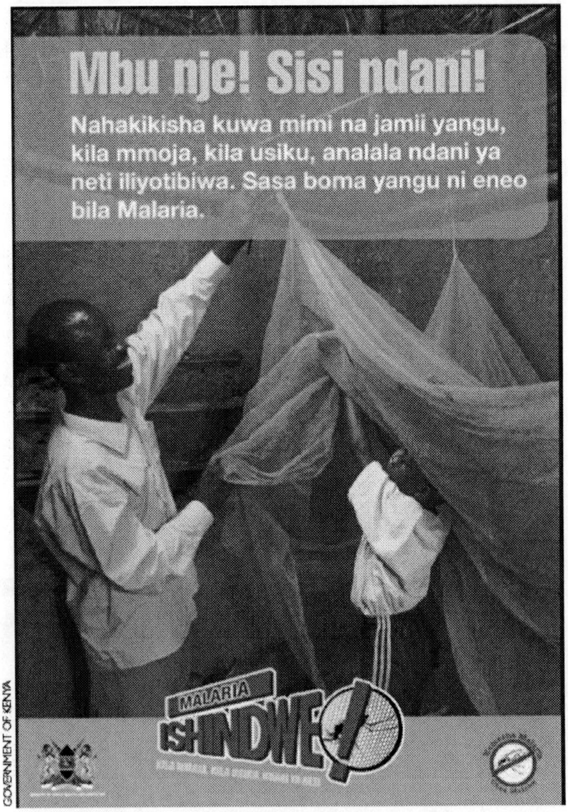

In this poster, which is part of a behavior change communication campaign encouraging year-round use of ITNs in Kenya, the father states, "I make sure that my family and I, everyone, every night, sleep inside a net. Now my homestead is malaria free." The campaign's theme is Everyone, Every Night, Inside the Net. PMI supports the use of similar behavior change communication materials to promote the consistent use of ITNs in all focus countries.

- In Tanzania, a year-long campaign was launched in early 2009 to distribute free ITNs to all children under five years of age with joint funding from PMI, The Global Fund to Fight AIDS, Tuberculosis and Malaria (Global Fund), the United Nations Children's Fund (UNICEF), the World Bank, and Malaria No More. By December 2009, more than 6 million net had been distributed in 10 regions. PMI contributed 1.8 million ITNs to this campaign and funded net distribution, training of supervisors and net distributors, and BCC activities before, during, and after the campaign. The BCC activities made use of a large network of community mobilizers to engage local residents on the importance of registering for and collecting their nets at distribution sites and using nets year round. A variety of print materials, road shows, school child-to-parent programs, and celebrity artists were used to support the mobilizers' work. In addition, a hang-up campaign used house-to-house visits to distribute brochures promoting year-round use of nets and helped family members hang their nets correctly.
- To achieve the **Liberian** NMCP's goal of universal net coverage (defined as one net per sleeping space, with a maximum of three sleeping spaces per household), PMI contributed 430,000 ITNs to a nationwide free net distribution campaign.

Sustaining High Coverage and Use through Routine ITN Distribution

Distribution of ITNs to achieve and sustain high net coverage in PMI countries involves both the public and private sectors. Many countries deliver ITNs through routine antenatal or immunization clinics, taking advantage of existing health services to reach the most vulnerable groups. Distribution through health facilities includes giving out free ITNs, selling ITNs at a highly subsidized price, and distributing vouchers that can be redeemed at private sector distribution points. The use of vouchers supports local retailers and strengthens the commercial market while reducing the burden on the public sector of handling the logistics of net distribution. Social marketing programs, which promote subsidized ITNs within the private sector or through community-based agents, have been used in several PMI countries, including Ghana, Madagascar, and Tanzania.

- Malawi plans to achieve universal coverage of ITNs through a multipronged approach to ITN distribution: routine distribution of free ITNs through antenatal and immunization clinics; periodic mass campaigns; and traditional social marketing through private sector outlets. During 2009, PMI procured nearly 1.8 million for distribution through antenatal and immunization clinics. PMI support has led to increased household ITN ownership and use by children under five. A population-based household survey in eight of Malawi's 28 districts in April 2009 showed that 59 percent percent of households owned one or more ITN and 61 percent of children under five had slept under an ITN the night before the survey. Integrating ITN distribution into the immunization program may help increase vaccination rates, and thus the overall health of young children.
- In Kenya, PMI procured 1.2 million ITNs for routine distribution through antenatal care and child welfare clinics to pregnant women and children under the age of one. While other distribution strategies are used in Kenya, including mass distribution, social marketing and commercial sales, this strategy ensures coverage of vulnerable groups and provides opportunities for interpersonal communication at the point of distribution, which increases net use.
- In Angola, during 2009, PMI supported the routine distribution of more than 412,000 free ITNs to pregnant women and children under five through clinics, as well as the sale of 9,700 subsidized and full-cost ITNs through social marketing outlets. PMI complemented this strategy by supporting a UNICEF-led integrated campaign in urban areas that included routine vaccinations, deworming, vitamin A distribution, and the distribution of 1.8 million ITNs to children under the age of one and pregnant women. PMI contributed nearly $1 million to support the purchase of nearly 92,000 ITNs and activities, such as logistics, monitoring, and BCC.

Achieving High Net Usage

While the number of ITNs distributed in sub-Saharan Africa has risen rapidly over the past several years, evidence from several countries continues to show gaps between net ownership and use (sleeping under a net every night). This has raised awareness of the need to expand and improve BCC efforts to instruct residents on proper hanging, use, and care of ITNs. BCC campaigns have included radio messages and talk shows, community mobilization events, video road shows, and interpersonal communication. Post campaign household visits to help and ensure their correct use is another that has been used successfully in several PMI focus countries.

In 2009, PMI supported BCC efforts to increase net usage in **Ghana** by training nearly 3,000 nongovernmental organization (NGO) staff, community leaders, and volunteers to deliver malaria campaign messages. An estimated 12.4 million residents were reached with malaria campaign messages through TV spots. Radio and community theater performances also played an important part of the PMI BCC program to increase net usage. Two radio campaigns reached 8 million people, and nearly 90,000 distribution through people attended community theater performances.

In Ethiopia, an assessment prior to the development of a comprehensive BCC strategy showed that net use was associated with a range of household and ITN-specific factors, including whether a house had been covered with whether an ITN had been received for free or purchased. To increase use of ITNs, PMI procured conical ITNs, which are more suitable to the traditional, round-shaped housing (tukuls) found in most rural areas of Ethiopia. This is being complemented by in-depth dissemination of information on four essential malaria actions, including through social ITN use, through a mix of BCC approaches.

Future Directions

Major achievements in increasing ITN coverage have been made in PMI countries during 2009, and many PMI countries have secured the resources to achieve universal coverage of populations at risk by the end of 2010; however, challenges remain:

- Resistance in Anopheles vector mosquitoes to pyrethroid insecticides used in ITNs has been reported, particularly in West Africa. Studies are under way to determine the impact of this resistance on the effectiveness of ITNs and to identify new insecticides for use in ITNs.
- Further studies of net durability and effectiveness are needed to determine the effective lifespan of long-lasting ITNs; early evidence indicates considerable differences among and even within countries.

- To maintain high levels of coverage, NMCPs will need hang nets properly to develop plans to replace expired nets with new ones. promising approach

For more information, please visit the ITN section of the PMI PMI website at

VOICES FROM THE FIELD

Universal ITN Coverage Campaign in Madagascar: Progress through Partnerships

In collaboration with UNICEF, the Global Fund, the International and Malagasy Red Cross, WHO, and the NMCP, PMI is supporting the 2009–2010 free mass distribution of ITNs to achieve universal coverage by the end of 2010 in Madagascar. In November and December 2009, with the help of local staff, community members and their leaders, about 1.7 million ITNs (1 million provided by PMI) were distributed to more than 820,000 households, protecting more than 4.1 million people in 19 health districts on the east coast of Madagascar, where malaria is endemic. Another 5.5 million ITNs (of which PMI is contributing 2.3 million) are planned for distribution during the last phase of the campaign in September–October 2010.

PMI involvement in the campaign was multifaceted: helping to develop the ITN program strategy; securing resources; serving on the planning committee; and developing monitoring tools to ensure that the campaign ran smoothly. When it became clear that PMI could not work directly with the Government of Madagascar due to the political situation in the country, PMI engaged the services of local faith-based organizations to distribute the nets at the community level.

Supervisory teams, deemed essential given the scope of the campaign and the difficulty of the terrain, were sent to all 19 districts covered by the campaign. Team members were drawn from all of the Roll Back Malaria partners involved in the campaign and included PMI staff and implementing partners. Supervisors were able to quickly resolve implementation problems in the field, ensuring that the campaign was able to reach the poorest and most vulnerable populations.

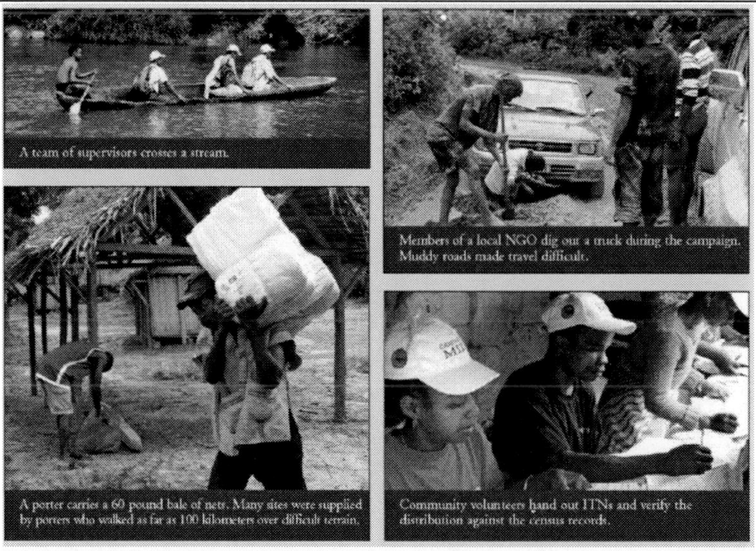

A team of supervisors crosses a stream.

Members of a local NGO dig out a truck during the campaign. Muddy roads made travel difficult.

A porter carries a 60 pound bale of nets. Many sites were supplied by porters who walked as far as 100 kilometers over difficult terrain.

Community volunteers hand out ITNs and verify the distribution against the census records.

2. PREVENTION – INDOOR RESIDUAL SPRAYING

> *"Malaria control is one of the best investments we have in global health ... We must build on successes wehave seen in places like Rwanda, Zambia and Zanzibar, where effective partnerships and proven tools, suchas insecticide-treated mosquito nets, spraying of homes with safe, effective insecticides, and malaria diagnosisand treatment have been used together to dramatically decrease deaths and illness."*
>
> – Rear Admiral R.T. Ziemer, USN (ret), U.S. Global Malaria Coordinator, December 15, 2009

Since 2006, PMI has been leading efforts to incorporate indoor residual spraying (IRS) with insecticides as a major component of malaria control efforts in Africa. Prior to the launch of PMI, IRS was being implemented by national malaria control programs (NMCPs) in only a few southern African countries and in Ethiopia and Eritrea, while the private sector was supporting spraying Ghana, and Zambia. In addition to building local capacity for IRS in the 15 focus countries, role, along with the World Health Organization (WHO) and other partners, in raising awareness of the value and feasibility of IRS as a malaria control measure in Africa.

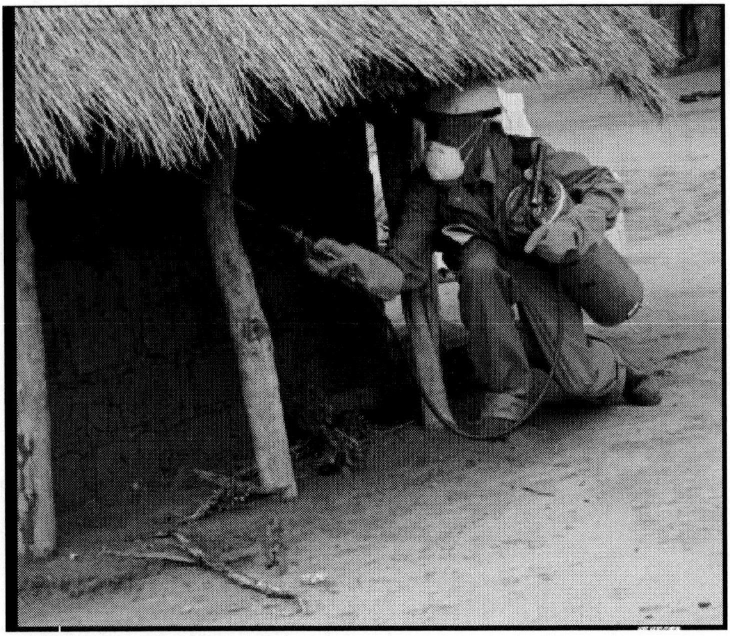

After spraying the inside of a home during an indoor residual spraying program in Uganda, as a final step, a spray operatorapplies insecticide on the eaves of a house, a major entryway for mosquitoes.

Indoor residual spraying consists of spraying the interior walls of homes with insecticides that remain effective from three to ten months, depending on the insecticide used, the type of wall surface, and whether the homeowner washes or replasters the wall after spraying. Malaria is transmitted by the bite of female Anopheles mosquitoes that are infected with malaria parasites. In Africa, these mosquitoes generally feed on people indoors at night and, after feeding, tend to rest on walls, where they can come into contact with the insecticide in sprayed homes. While the insecticides used for IRS may have some repellent effect, the greatest impact of IRS is killing mosquitoes before they transmit malaria parasites to another person. As a result, IRS provides community- level, rather than individual, protection. In order for an IRS program to be fully effective, WHO recommends that at least 80 percent of houses in a targeted area be sprayed usually once or twice a year, depending on the length of the transmission season and the duration of effectiveness of the insecticide.

PMI IRS Summary

During 2009, more than 26 million people were protected through PMI-supported IRS operations in the 15 PMI focus countries (see table below). To conduct these IRS operations, PMI supported the training of more than 21,000 spray personnel, who sprayed more than 6.6 PMI has played a key million houses.

IRS Coverage Rates

The PMI target for its IRS activities is for 85 percent of all houses in the targeted geographic areas to be spraye As part of each round of spraying, houses targeted for spraying are counted, and coverage is calculated ba on the percentage of those houses that were successfully sprayed. IRS rounds supported by PMI have consistently reached, and in most cases exceeded, the 85 percent coverage target. During 2009, coverage rates for PMI- supported spray rounds ranged from 88 to 99 percent, illustrating the remarkably high acceptance rate of IRS by communities.

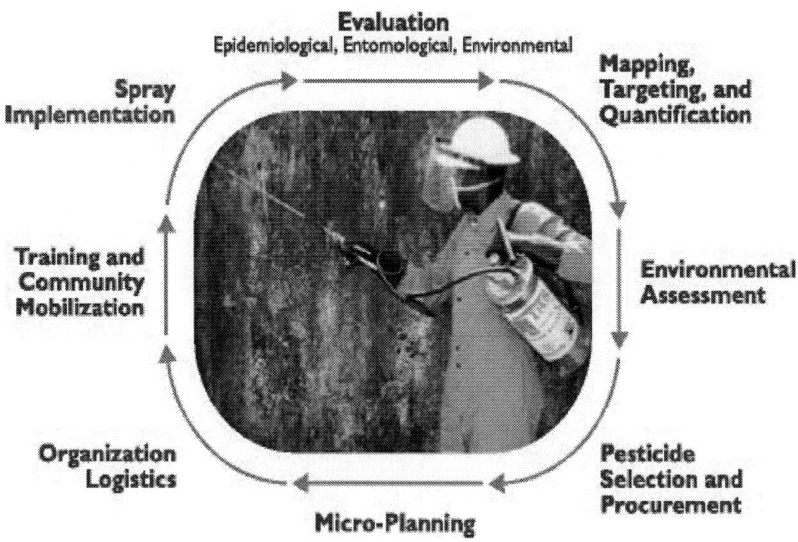

Figure 1. IRS Management Cycle.

Managing IRS

Indoor residual spraying programs present numerous logistical and operational challenges. Spray operations can involve many hundreds of spray operators and supervisors, plus clinicians, community mobilizers and educators, environmental officers, drivers, warehouse staff, and office workers. Depending on the type of insecticide used, soak pits or evaporation tanks and wash facilities must be constructed to meet environmental regulations. A fleet of vehicles is required to transport the spray teams, insecticide, and equipment to the targeted areas. Local residents must be willing to cooperate with the spray teams and permit access to their homes by removing furniture that could limit spraying of all wall surfaces, and then replacing those items within the house after waiting two hours for the walls to dry. Additionally, IRS operations must occur within a narrow timeframe, immediately preceding or at the start of the rainy season, to ensure maximum protection during the malaria transmission season (see Figure 1, above).

PMI IRS SUMMARY TABLE				
Indicator[1,2]	**PMIYear1 (2006)**	**PMIYear2 (2007)**	**PMIYear3 (2008)**	**PMIYear4 (2009)**
People protected by IRS	2,097,056	18,827,709	25,157,408	26,965,164
Spray personnel trained[3]	1,336	13,795	19,077	21,664
Houses sprayed	414,456	4,353,747	6,101,271	6,656,524

[1] The numbers reported in this table are up-to-date as of January 1, 2010, and include all 15 PMI focus countries. In addition, during 2009, the USG provided support for an IRS campaign in Zimbabwe that protected 929,600 people. For data by country, see Appendix 2.

[2] A cumulative count of the number of people trained, people protected, houses targeted, and houses sprayed for Years 1 through 4 of PMI is not provided since some areas have been sprayed on more than one occasion.

[3] Spray personnel are defined as spray operators, supervisors, and ancillary personnel. These calculations do not include many people trained to conduct infor-mation and community mobilization programs surrounding IRS campaigns.

The PMI-supported IRS program in Rwanda, which enjoys strong political support at both the district and national levels and significant participation from community political leaders, health workers, and others, provides a good example of the complexity and scope of an IRS campaign. In 2009, PMI supported two rounds of spraying. During the second round, the NMCP trained 4,450 local residents as community mobilizers who went house to house, encouraging residents to cooperate with the IRS program and prepare for the spray teams. Nearly 2,300 community members, nearly half of whom were women (pregnant women were excluded), were hired and trained as spray operators. IRS teams identified 302,000 houses for spraying and succeeded in spraying 98 percent of them, protecting more than 1.3 million residents. The advantage of using local residents for these tasks is that by working within their own communities they are better able to explain the benefits of IRS to their neighbors and to adjust spray schedules to accommodate their neighbors' needs.

Working with NMCPs

PMI's level of involvement in IRS programs varies depending on the needs of the focus country. Zambia is an example of a country where the Ministry of Health and the NMCP take primary responsibility for strategic planning, resource mobilization, provision of staff, coordination of training, and procurement and distribution of commodities for the IRS program. The health districts produce micro-plans and implement spray operations. PMI provides insecticides, spray pumps, and personal protective equipment in 15 of the 36 IRS districts in the country, training of spray operators in all 36 districts, development of IRS technical guidelines, general technical support to improve the overall management and implementation of the Zambian IRS program, and technical assistance to promote compliance with environmental and human safeguards.

In countries where IRS has not been used for many years, PMI provides management and implementation responsibility for the IRS program, while gradually building capacity within the NMCP. For example, in Benin, upon the request of the NMCP, PMI supported the development of a long-term IRS strategy that will guide future IRS operations. PMI also supports capacity building within NMCPs related to insecticide resistance and environmental management.

Capacity Building for IRS

Building local capacity is a critical component of all IRS programs that receive PMI support. PMI has developed a capacity and sustainability tracking tool that lists the key activities involved in an IRS program, including planning, entomological surveillance, environmental compliance, and training of spray personnel. As successive spray rounds are implemented, PMI tracks its national and local counterparts' progress toward assuming responsibility for IRS activities.

For example, in Ghana, Liberia, and Ethiopia, PMI improved the skills of local technicians to carry out entomological monitoring related to IRS through training and rehabilitated the laboratories they work in. In Ethiopia and Zambia, capacity has been strengthened for environmental monitoring and compliance that will ensure that IRS programs there are safe and well managed. In Ethiopia, this included creating insecticide storage facilities at the district level and training local personnel who are involved in handling insecticides, so they are well versed in the proper procedures to prevent or mitigate any negative health or environmental effects from IRS. And, in Zambia, as a result of PMI's work on strengthening the Ministry of Tourism, Environment and Natural Resources is now heading environmental assessment activities.

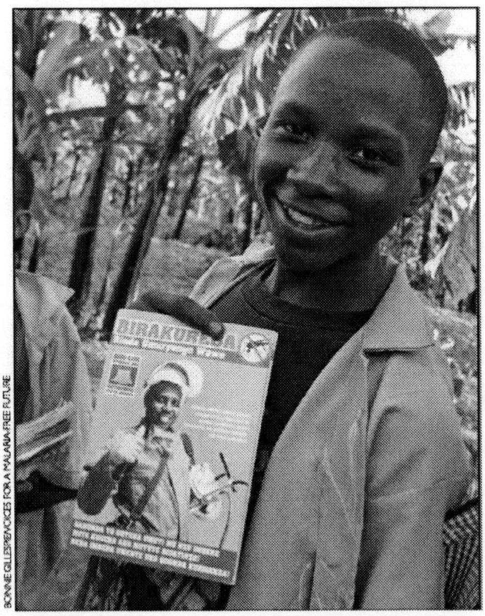

In Rwanda, a young man hands out a flier for an IRS campaign. Information and social mobilization efforts serve a critical role in gaining the participation of community members in IRS programs.

Insecticide Resistance

Insecticide resistance is emerging as a major threat to both IRS and insecticide-treated nets across Africa. Resistance to one or more types of insecticides is of particular concern in West African countries, including Benin and Ghana, as well as in the East African countries of Ethiopia and Uganda. Selection pressure for insecticide resistance can come from both agricultural and public health use of insecticides. PMI is working closely with WHO and other partners to develop more robust resistance monitoring and mitigation strategies. In addition, several new formulations of insecticides are under development, and it is hoped that they will soon be however, it can be expected that resistance will appear for each new insecticide that is developed. For this reason, PMI will continue to work with partners, including other U.S. Government agencies, such as the Environmental Protection Agency and the Department of Agriculture, and focus countries' governmental agencies and insecticide manufacturers to promote the judicious use of insecticides.

In the Oromia Region of Ethiopia, PMI provided comprehensive support to monitor insecticide susceptibility. This included carrying out insecticide susceptibility tests, training staff, procuring needed materials, and analyzing data. Ethiopia has a long history of DDT use for IRS, and the recent PMI-supported susceptibility testing of mosquitoes to a range of insecticides showed that there was resistance to DDT. Following these findings, the Government of Ethiopia, in collaboration with WHO and PMI, expanded insecticide resistance monitoring to the remainder of the country, confirming the findings observed in Oromia. This has led to a change in the class of insecticide used for IRS in Oromia as well as in the rest of the country.

Another insecticide resistance challenge relates to building local capacity for the optimal use of insecticides, so NMCPs can decide how, when, and where to deploy IRS. PMI is working with WHO to promote "integrated vector management," which is defined as "a rational decision- making process for optimal use of resources for vector control." For IRS, this involves building capacity for entomologic monitoring to guide insecticide selection and the targeting and timing of IRS applications. PMI Zambia, is linking NMCPs with national health research institutes national capacity, the and universities, such as the Noguchi Memorial Institute for Medical Research in Ghana and the Malaria Research and Training Center in Mali, to provide the necessary training and technical support.

Environmental Management of Insecticides

All IRS activities supported by PMI adhere to U.S. Government and international regulations and treaties regarding the safe storage, transport, use, and disposal of insecticides. These regulations ensure that development programs using pesticides, such as PMI, are not only economically sustainable, but also protect the host country's residents, vector control workers, and environment.

Insecticide management is relatively new to most ministries of health in Africa. For that reason, PMI is working with those ministries, as well as with focus countries' available for IRS. Over time, ministries of agriculture and the environment, to build capacity and create awareness of the need for safe management of insecticides in compliance with international regulations. For example, in 2009, PMI worked with the Government of Zambia to improve the national IRS program's compliance with human and environmental safeguards. With PMI's support, Zambia sprayed more than 1 million homes in 36 districts in 2009 and protected people.

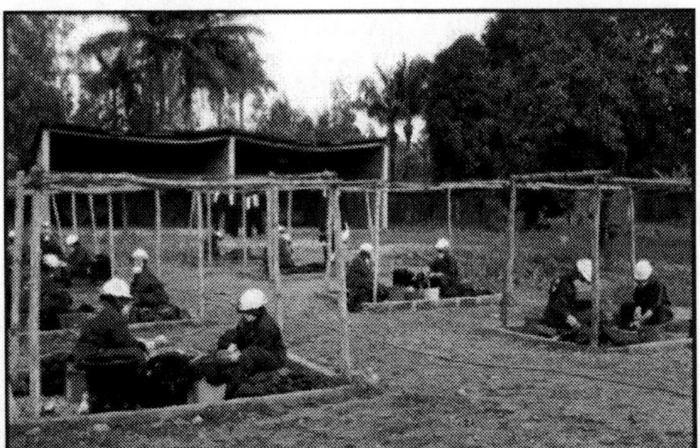

LAURA MCGORMAN/PMI

Following an IRS spraying program in Benin, women wash the sprayers' personal protective clothing. Water from this operation and from cleaning spray pumps is handled according to U.S. Government, international, and host country environmental regulations.

To meet the environmental requirements of such a large program, PMI assisted the NMCP in constructing evaporation tanks and soak pits for disposal of waste; performing before, during, and post-spraying compliance inspections in 15 districts; and collecting samples for environmental monitoring of DDT. In addition, PMI provided technical support to the Environmental Council of Zambia to undertake a national strategic environmental assessment for the expanding national IRS program.

PMI is also working with WHO and others, including insecticide manufacturers, to develop IRS management practices that could serve as models for programs beyond PMI focus countries. These practices cover a range of environmental considerations, from stock management and control to worker and resident safety.

Working with Partners

Since the Initiative began, PMI has collaborated with private sector IRS programs, notably in Ghana, Malawi, and Zambia. PMI also works with the Global Business Coalition for HIV/AIDS, TB, and Malaria to strengthen links between the private sector and NMCPs, particularly as it relates to IRS and vector control.

- In Ghana, the PMI-supported program has benefited from assistance and collaboration from the AngloGold Ashanti mining company, which has conducted an IRS program since 2005 (see Voices from the Field on page 22).

- In Malawi, where PMI has been partnering withDwangwa Sugar Estates in Nkhotakota District since2007, operations expanded to cover the whole district,nearly 75,000 houses, in 2009. Lessons learned fromthe previous two spray rounds were used to improvethe overall quality of spray operations.
- In Zambia, the Mopane and Konkola Copper Minesand the Zambia Sugar Company have been activeprivate sector partners in the NMCP IRS program,which is also supported by PMI. The mining compa-nies procured the insecticides, spray pumps, personalprotective equipment, and supported operational costsin areas where their workers and dependents live. Theyalso provided storage for IRS commodities. In 2009,the two copper mines sprayed 52,680 structures, andPMI supported the spraying of 1.1 million houses.

PMI also collaborates with multilateral and nongovern-mental organizations.For example, following the coup more than 6 million d'état in Madagascar in March 2009, PMI was unable to work directly with government ministries, but continued to collaborate with the Global Fund to ensure the 2009 national IRS campaign would go forward to cover more than 1.2 million houses and protect more than 6.7 million people. PMI supported spraying of 216,000 houses, protecting more than 1.2 million people. PMI also worked with the Malagasy Red Cross, which carried out community-level activities, such as community mobilization; information, education, and communication; and the actual spraying.

Future Directions

The last few years have seen a renewed recognition of the importance of IRS as part of comprehensive malaria control programs in Africa. As malaria prevalence decreases, PMI will support countries as they adjust their malaria control programs. For example, on Zanzibar, where malaria prevalence has decreased markedly, the malaria strategy has shifted away from annual IRS operations and instead relies on focal spraying when an outbreak is and Zambia. PMI also detected, in addition to diagnosing and treating malaria Coalition for HIV/AIDS, cases in health facilities and maintaining high ITN usage.

VOICES FROM THE FIELD

Collaboration in IRS Scale-Up in Ghana

With a patchwork of IRS programs across a diverse landscape, Ghana is undertaking an ambitious scale-up of IRS for malaria control. The program is based on a four-way collaboration among the Government of Ghana, the private mining company AngloGold Ashanti (AGA) and PMI, and with significant financial support from the Global Fund.

In the southern forest zone, AGA has conducted malaria control operations in Obuasi District since 2005. AGA's well regarded program has focused on IRS and targeted larviciding, but also has supported a scale-up of ITNs and ACTs. A 75 percent reduction in malaria was recorded in the company's workforce between 2005 and 2008.

In the northern savannah zone, the PM I-supported program, which is implemented in collaboration with the Ghana Health Service (GHS), covered six contiguous districts and reached more than 708,000 people in 2009; two more districts will be added in 2010. PMI's program has been characterized by a strongly collaborative approach.

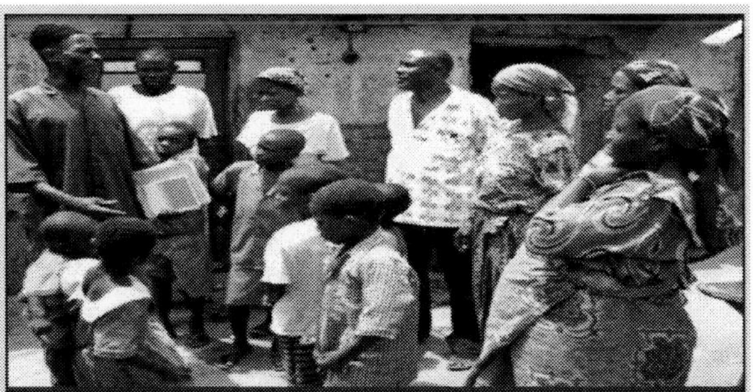

In Karaga, Ghana, a community mobilizer talks with a family about an upcoming IRS program and the spray schedule for the area. In Ghana, coverage rates averaged more than 90 percent, reflecting communities' support for IRS.

Community mobilizers rely upon existing GHS health volunteer networks and have enjoyed the full support of the area's traditional leaders. Spray operators are recruited from local communities with the help of GHS. Entomologic monitoring is conducted in collaboration with the University of Ghana and GHS Northern Region staff. AGA has provided valuable assistance in such areas as community sensitization, training of trainers, and training of spray operators in the field. Monitoring visits have been conducted by the NMCP and the Ghanaian Environmental Protection Agency staff from Accra and the regional capital, Tamale.

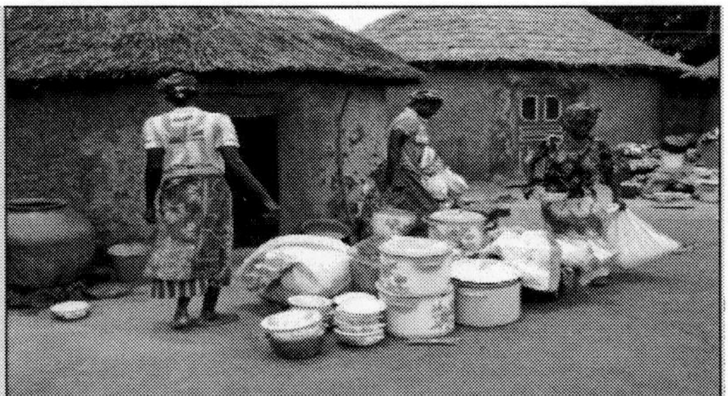

To prepare for spraying, women empty their homes of their possessions to allow the sprayers to have access to their interior walls. Once the walls have dried, which usually takes two hours, the women will be able to move their belongings back into their homes.

Ghana's national malaria control strategy calls for a scale-up of IRS to one-third of the country's 138 districts. To this end, Ghana, with assistance from PMI, WHO, and AGA, was recommended to receive a Global Fund grant in October 2009 for implementation of IRS in 35 additional districts by 2013, with AGA as the grant's Principal Recipient. PMI's logistics experience will be valuable to AGA as it begins to set up its operations far from the company's mining facilities and in regions with a vast, challenging terrain.

3. PREVENTION – MALARIA IN PREGNANCY

"The key to saving lives, especially children's lives, is to expand proven approaches and interventionsuntil they reach each and every pregnant woman and child who needs them."

– Rear Admiral R.T. Ziemer, USN (ret), U.S. Global Malaria Coordinator, October 6, 2009

Malaria infection during pregnancy poses a serious health risk to both the mother and her unborn child. Prevention and treatment of malaria in pregnant women depend on a combination of measures, including the use of long-lasting insecticide-treated nets (ITNs), intermittent preventive treatment for pregnant women (IPTp), and prompt diagnosis and effective treatment when malaria infections are detected.

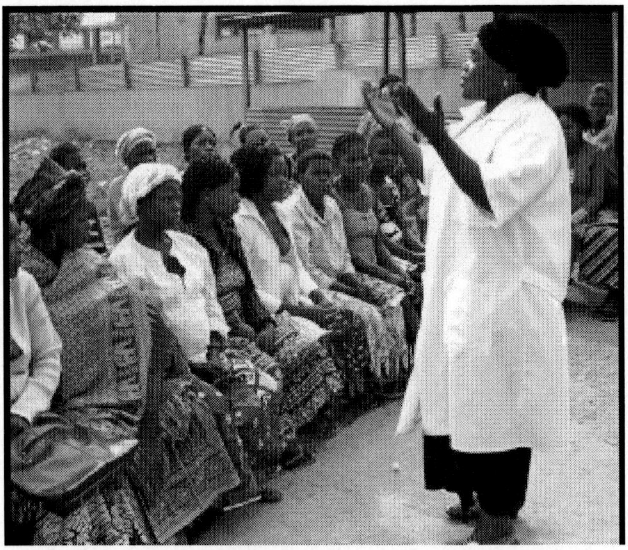

A health worker presents information to pregnant women during a malaria awareness workshop at a health facilityin Uige, Angola. With PMI's support, pregnant women are encouraged to attend antenatal clinics to receive atleast two doses of IPTp.

Intermittent preventive treatment for pregnant women is a highly effective means of reducing the serious conse-quences of malaria in both the pregnant woman and her unborn child, which include maternal anemia and low birthweight babies. IPTp consists of the administration of at least two doses of the antimalarial drug, sulfadox-ine-pyrimethamine (SP), given not less than one month apart during the second and third trimesters of pregnancy. Since more than 70 percent of pregnant women attend antenatal clinics at least once during their pregnancies in most African countries, IPTp is administered during routine antenatal clinic visits. It has been estimated that IPTp alone could prevent 75,000 to 200,000 infant deaths each year in Africa. IPTp also benefits maternal health by reducing anemia in the third trimester.

PMI Malaria in Pregnancy Summary

Most supplies of SP for IPTp are provided by national governments or other donors, so PMI has focused its efforts increasing IPTp coverage rates by:

- Training health care workers in malaria in pregnancy (MIP) and focused antenatal care (FANC) – a comprehensive package of antenatal care services;
- Strengthening supply chain management systems to deliver and track commodities;
- Providing behavior change communications at the community level to promote early attendance at antenatal clinics and uptake of IPTp and nightly use of ITNs; and
- Identifying and working to lift cultural barriers that prevent women from accessing malaria prevention and treatment services.

Since its launch in 2005, PMI has procured more than 4 million IPTp treatments (see table below). In 2009 alone, PMI procured 1.6 million IPTp treatments and supported training for more than 14,000 health workers on control of malaria during pregnancy, usually within the context of FANC. Additionally, in 2009, PMI procured more than 15 million ITNs and assisted with the distribution of another 2.9 million ITNs – procured by other donors – through antenatal clinics and mass distribution campaigns.

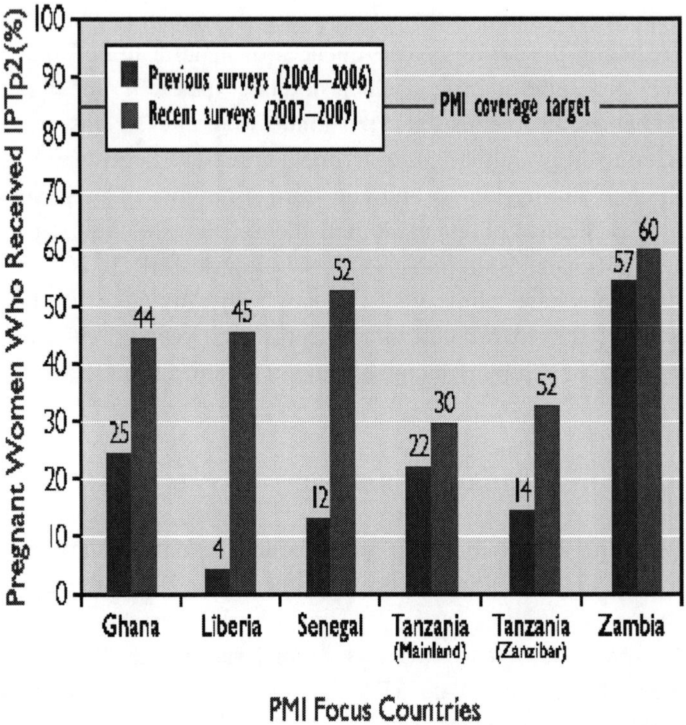

Notes: (1) The countries included in this graph are those PMI focus countries for which there are two data points from nation-wide household surveys for the indicator. (2) IPTp2 is defined as at least two doses of SP during the last pregnancy, with at least one given during an antenatal clinic visit.

Figure 1. Increases in IPTp2 Rates in Selected PMI Countries.

IPTp Coverage Rates

The PMI IPTp coverage target is 85 percent or above for two doses of IPTp across the 15 PMI focus countries. Many challenges stand in the way of achieving this target. While the proportion of pregnant women who have received at least one IPTp dose during their last pregnancy has increased rapidly across Africa since 2004–2005, coverage with two or more IPTp doses (IPTp2) has increased much more slowly. In spite of this, several PMI countries have reported encouraging results. For example, nationwide surveys showed that IPTp2 increased from 25 to 44 percent in Ghana, from 4 to 45 percent in Liberia, and from 12 to 52 percent in Senegal between 2005–2006 and 2008–2009 (see Figure 1, above).

PMI MALARIA IN PREGNANCY SUMMARY TABLE					
Indicator[1]	PMIYear[1] (2006)	PMIYear[2] (2007)	PMIYear[3] (2008)	PMIYear[4] (2009)	Cumulative
IPTp treatments procured[2]	-	1,349,999	1,018,333	1,657,998	4,026,330 (3,524,122 distributed)
Health workers trained in IPTp[4]	1,994	3,153	12,557	14,015	N/A[3]

[1] The numbers reported in this table are up-to-date as of January 1, 2010, and include all 15 PMI focus countries. In addition, during 2009, the USG provided support for malaria in pregnancy activities in the Democratic Republic of Congo, Nigeria, and Sudan; more than 700 health workers were trained in IPTp and 430,000 IPTp treatments were procured and distributed. For data by country, see Appendix 2.

[2] Most countries' SP needs for IPTp are met by national governments and other donors.

[3] A cumulative count of individual health workers trained for Years 1 through 4 of PMI is not provided since some health workers have been trained on more than one occasion.

[4] IPTp is usually given as part of a larger package of focused antenatal care services.

Integrating Malaria into Maternal Health Programs

PMI supports activities to prevent and treat malaria in pregnancy within the context of broader reproductive health services across the 15 focus countries. Most African countries have adopted FANC for the care of women during their pregnancy and the postpartum period. The objective of FANC is to ensure that antenatal care visits include health promotion and disease prevention activities, early detection and treatment of the complications of pregnancy and diseases, birth preparedness, and complication readiness. PMI has supported the scale-up of FANC in many countries, in several cases in partnership with the U.S. President's Emergency Plan for AIDS Relief (PEPFAR) and the U.S. Agency for International Development (USAID) maternal and child health programs, by funding pre-service and in-service training of health workers, supportive supervision, job aids, and improved supply chain management of key commodities. For example:

- In Ethiopia, both PMI and PEPFAR have impleactivities that have increased prevention and treatment of malaria using a range of different approaches, including community discussions, radio listening groups, school malaria clubs, and mass media. With

PEPFAR support, PMI's community-based, malaria-specific BCC interventions are delivered at 48 sites that aim to increase antenatal clinic attendance and prevention of mother-to-child transmission of HIV.

- Since it began work in Tanzania, PMI has been working with both Mainland Tanzania and Zanzibar's ministries of health and social welfare to strengthen MIP programs at the district level. The objective of the program is to increase uptake of IPTp by improving the quality of antenatal care services through FANC; regular supervision of health workers; and strengthened supply chain management for critical commodities, such as SP, iron, and ITN vouchers at the district level. A major thrust of the program is to ensure that all antenatal programs on the Tanzania Mainland and Zanzibar have at least one provider trained in FANC/MIP and that all districts have ongoing supportive supervision. With PMI support, through a "cascade" training program, at least four FANC trainers were trained in each of the 133 districts on the Mainland, and 24 trainers were developed for Zanzibar. They in turn trained a total of 2,000 health workers in FANC on the Mainland and 288 on Zanzibar during 2009. Altogether, 60 percent of antenatal care facilities on the Mainland and 67 percent of those on Zanzibar now have FANC-trained providers.
- In Uganda, PMI works with the business community to improve access to and usage of a broad range of health services by company employees, their dependents, and the surrounding community. Services include treatment for malaria, tuberculosis, HIV/AIDS, family planning, and reproductive health for company employees. The program is supported by both PMI and PEPFAR and uses a cost-sharing approach with local businesses to procure and distribute ITNs and to provide clean water and cups for directly observed IPTp, BCC materials and activities, and supportive supervision for health clinic staff. In 2009, this program worked with 11 large private companies in Uganda and distributed nearly 46,000 SP treatments and 100,000 free ITNs to pregnant women.

Improving Clarity of IPTp Guidelines

In the past, most national IPTp guidelines required that IPTp be administered at specific weeks of gestation.

Since many women may not know the date of conception and tend to make their first antenatal visit later than recommended, these guidelines have caused confusion among health workers who tried to calculate the correct timing for IPTp treatments. PMI has supported revision of country IPTp guidelines to improve their clarity and simplicity. **Malawi** was one of the first countries to adopt these changes to its IPTp policy.

With PMI support, Malawi has also addressed other causes of the low uptake of the second dose of IPTp by disseminating gestational wheels, which indicate the week of gestation (based on the presumed date of conception) and simplify the timing of IPTp dosages, providing cups and safe water vessels to aid directly observed therapy, and developing BCC materials for both staff and patients to increase understanding of the importance of receiving two doses of IPTp. To encourage women to attend antenatal clinics for the recommended number of visits and at the appropriate times during pregnancy, PMI launched a BCC campaign at the community level using small grants to eight community-based and nongovernmental organizations, and at the national level using radio and other mass media. Following these changes, a random household survey in eight of the country's 28 districts showed that IPTp2 rates had increased from 48 to 69 percent.

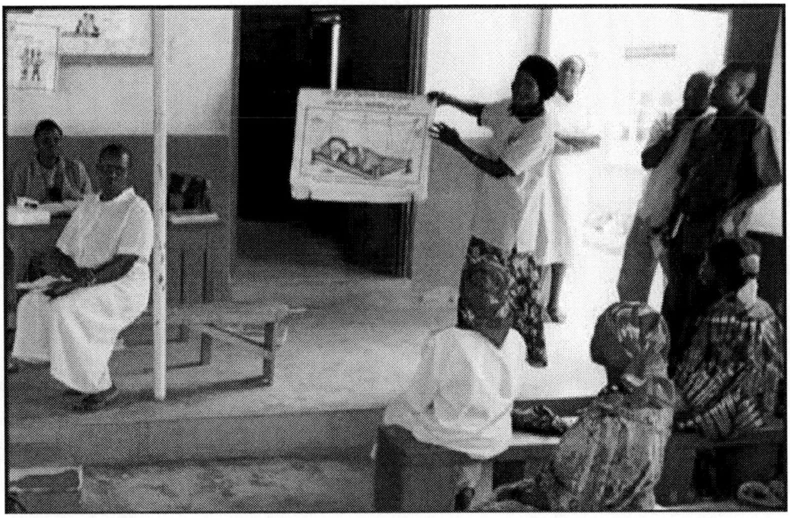

PHILIP BOWEN/MIHV

In Koboko Health Center in Uganda, Ayite Matata, who works with the Uganda Malaria Communities Program, delivers a malaria health talk about the importance of using an ITN during and after pregnancy.

Overcoming Cultural Barriers to IPTp

In many African countries, women hide their pregnancies for cultural reasons until they become visibly pregnant. As a result, they are often late in seeking antenatal care, which makes it difficult to complete the recommended two IPTp doses. PMI has been working to reduce cultural barriers to early antenatal clinic attendance andIPTp. For example, in Mali, PMI has opened a dialoguewith more than 950 religious leaders on pregnancy andthe risks of malaria during pregnancy and what familiescan do to reduce those risks (see Voices from the Fieldon page 28).

In Zambia, a 2008 assessment in the two provinces thathad the lowest reported IPTp rates in the last nationwidehousehold survey showed that a woman's decision to seekantenatal care is heavily influenced by her father or malepartner, who rarely attend antenatal clinics and do notreceive crucial educational messages that accompanythose services. To increase IPTp utilization, PMI isworking with women's groups to educate men about theneed for antenatal care and the prevention of malariaduring pregnancy.

Supply Chain Management Challenges

Although SP costs only $0.10 per treatment and is relatively easy to administer as a single dose, weak pharmaceutical management systems in most African countries are limiting progress toward meeting IPTp targets. Since SP needs in most of the 15 PMI focus countries are already being met by the host government or other donors, PMI has focused its efforts on strengthening supply chain management systems to forecast drug needs, monitor stock levels, and respond quickly to potential stockouts.

In Zambia, PMI supported a quantification exercise for SP in 2009 that showed that a stockout was imminent due to delays in SP procurements and inappropriate use of that drug for the treatment of acute malarial illnesses. To resolve this problem, PMI procured 2 million SP tablets through its Central Emergency Procurement Fund and provided pharmaceutical system strengthening support to prevent SP stockouts from reoccurring.

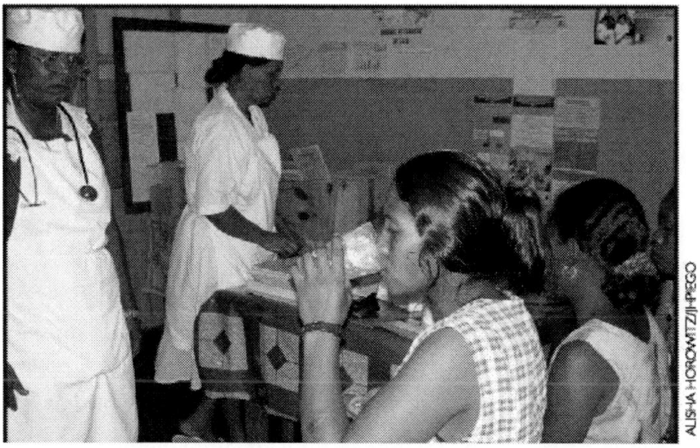

An expectant mother takes her first dose of IPTp at the Brickaville, Madagascar, antenatal clinic under the watchful eye of a midwife. PMI supports behavior change communication activities that promote regular antenatal clinic attendance.

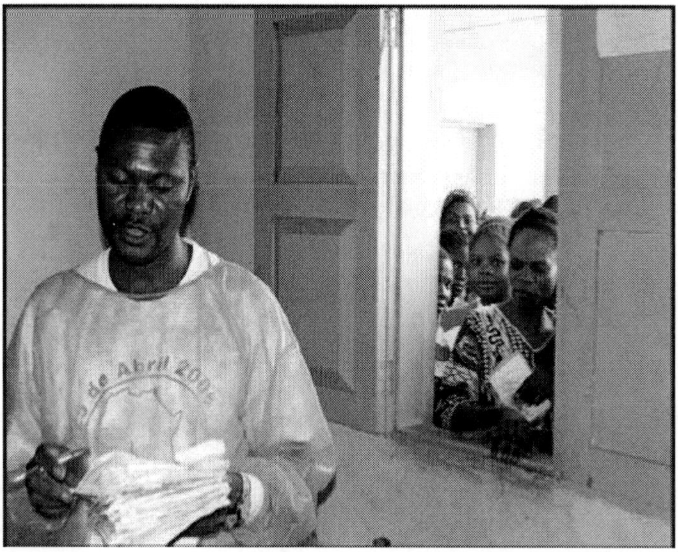

While a clinician reviews their papers, women wait to receive a free ITN at an antenatal clinic in Kuimba, Angola. PMI uses free distribution of ITNs through antenatal clinics to attract greater numbers of pregnant women to the clinics.

Parasite Resistance to SP

Sulfadoxine-pyrimethamine is the only antimalarial drug approved by the World Health Organization for IPTp, but its efficacy, as measured by treatment success in children under five, is declining in many African countries. IPTp efficacy trials in sub-Saharan Africa showed that two doses of IPTp with SP continued to provide substantial benefits to women in areas with SP resistance levels as high as 50 percent in children under five. For this reason, the World Health Organization has recommended that in areas of moderate to high, stable malaria transmission, countries that are already implementing IPTp with SP continue to do so and evaluate SP effectiveness. PMI is currently supporting operations research studies in **Malawi**, **Mali**, **Uganda**, and **Zambia** to better understand whether parasite resistance to SP in pregnant women is associated with any decrease in effectiveness of IPTp.

Future Directions

IPTp is currently only recommended in areas of moderate to high malaria transmission. As countries scale up their malaria prevention and treatment measures and malaria prevalence falls, PMI will assist NMCPs with periodic reassessments of their IPTp policies. For example, on **Zanzibar**, where the prevalence of malaria in the general population is less than 1 percent, PMI is supporting studies to guide policies on malaria in pregnancy. At the same time, PMI will help NMCPs place greater emphasis on the use of ITNs by pregnant women and their infant children and on the detection and prompt treatment of malaria infections.

VOICES FROM THE FIELD

Malian Religious Leaders Take an Active Role in Prevention of Malaria during Pregnancy

Imam Zeidy Drame of Omar Ben Katab Mosque in Lafiabougou, in the southern quarters of Bamako, Mali, is concerned about the negative impact of malaria on pregnant women in his community. He learned about the dangers of malaria through a PM I-supported program that works with more than 950 traditional and religious leaders to lift barriers that prevent women from accessing antenatal care services early in their pregnancies. These leaders are part of an interfaith health promotion network in Mali called *Réseau des Leaders Religieux pour la Promotion de la Santé*. The network encourages Muslim and Christian leaders to use their weekly sermons or teachings to promote openness in talking about pregnancy.

Since many Malians believe that talking about a pregnancy before it is visible can bring bad luck, women tend to hide their pregnancy and do not make their first antenatal clinic visit until late in their pregnancies. With PMI support, these leaders are trying to change this practice through teachings based on passages from the Koran and Bible and by educating and encouraging dialogue among couples about malaria and pregnancy.

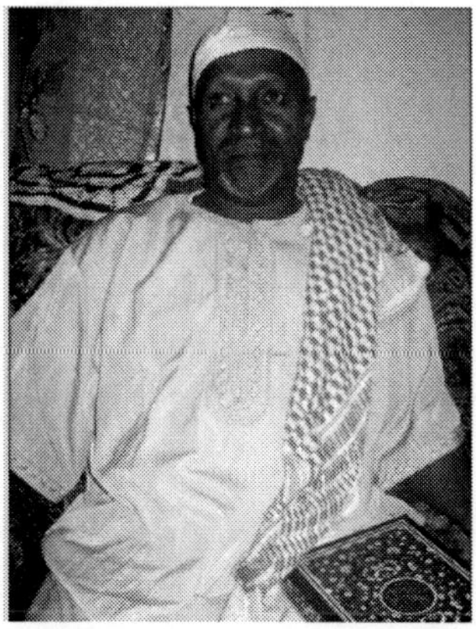

Imam Zeidy Drame of the Omar Ben Katab Mosque in Lafiabougou, Mali, uses teachings from the Koran to encourage pregnant women to attend antenatal care clinics and receive IPTp to reduce the risk of malaria in pregnancy.

PMI is working with the *Réseau des Leaders Religieux* to develop advocacy and training materials for use by other religious leaders. The materials, which include a standard sermon for Friday prayers, use clear and simple words to describe the risks of malaria for a pregnant woman and her newborn child and discuss cultural barriers to taking IPTp. Armed with teachings from the Koran and with an increased understanding of the dangers of malaria in pregnant women and young children, Imam Drame now preaches that "Islam encourages us to use all the resources available to us to prevent disease and preserve our health" and that men should communicate with their spouse on health matters.

4. Case Management – Diagnosis and Treatment

"We know we can put an end to this cycle of disease and poverty. In the last few years, we have witnessed a growingglobal effort to combat this curable and preventable disease. We are using proven drugs to treat malarial illness andsimple tools to prevent the disease, including insecticide nets, indoor spraying, and safe, inexpensive drugs for pregnantwomen. Millions of people have benefited, translating to lives saved and the advancement of human progress."

– U.S. Secretary of State Hillary Clinton, World Malaria Day celebration, April 24, 2009

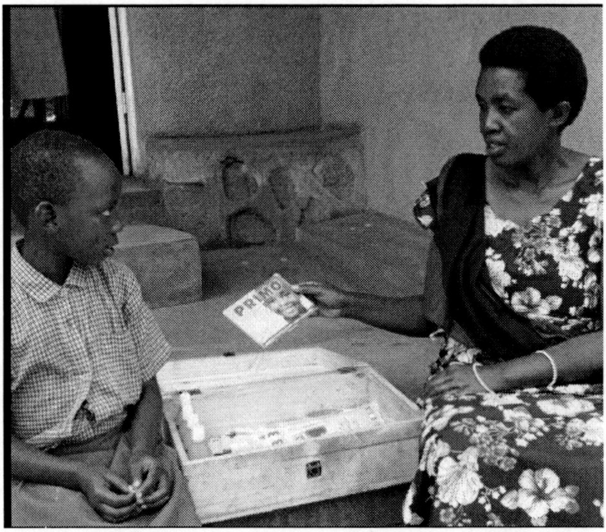

A community health worker and a young boy in Rwanda discuss the importance of taking the proper doses of anti-malarial drugs. In Rwanda, PRIMO, a branded artemisinin-based combination therapy, is used for community-basedmanagement of fever and is available in licensed private sector shops. PRIMO comes in a special package with easy-to-understand, illustrated instructions to ensure that children receive the correct dose and take the full treatment regimen.

Artemisinin-based combination therapies (ACTs) are the recommended first-line treatment for uncomplicated *P. falciparum* malaria in most malaria-affected regions of Africa. Effective case management of malaria depends on early, accurate diagnosis and prompt treatment with an effective drug. In 2009, the World Health Organization (WHO) issued updated guidelines for malaria case management that recommend that all people with suspected malaria undergo confirmatory testing for malaria parasites with good quality microscopy or rapid diagnostic tests (RDTs) before they receive treatment. This change in guidance was based on concerns that overuse of ACTs might promote the spread of drug resistance. In addition, as the incidence of malaria falls with the scale-up of effective control measures, an increasing percentage of people with fever will not have malaria infections and will need to be correctly diag-nosed and treated for other conditions.

Besides being highly effective antimalarial drugs, ACTs may reduce the probability of the emergence of drug-resistant malaria parasites, and thus prolong the effective lifetimes of the individual drugs. Since ACTs cost several times more than traditional first-line malaria treatments, such as chloroquine or sulfadoxine-pyrimethamine (SP), and have a much shorter shelf-life of just 18 to 24 months, accurate forecasting of drug needs and good pharmaceuti- cal management are critical to the effective use of ACTs.

PMI Case Management Summary

During 2009, across the 15 PMI focus countries, PMI procured more than 29 million ACT treatments (see table below). PMI also assisted with the distribution of more than 8 million ACTs that were procured by other donors. During 2009, more than 41,000 health workers were trained in the correct use of ACTs. To improve diagnostic testing of malaria, PMI purchased 6 million RDTs and, in 2009 alone, funded the training of more than 2,800 laboratory staff in microscopic and RDT diagnosis. PMI also supports the purchase of drugs for treating severe malaria and training of health workers on recognizing and managing severe malaria.

Case Management Coverage Rates

PMI's case management coverage targets are:

- 85 percent of children under five with suspected malaria will have received ACT treatment within 24 hours of the onset of symptoms; and
- 85 percent of governmental health facilities will have ACTs available for treatment of uncomplicated malaria.

PMI CASE MANAGEMENT SUMMARY TABLE						
Indicator[1]		PMIYear[1] (2006)	PMIYear[2] (2007)	PMIYear[3] (2008)	PMIYear[4] (2009)	Cumulative
Treatment	ACT treatments procured	1,229,550	11,537,433	15,454,709	29,616,342	57,838,034 (40,113,517 distributed)
	ACT treatments procured by other partners and distributed by PMI	-	8,709,140	112,330	8,855,401	17,676,871
	Health workers trained in use of ACTs	8,344	20,864	35,397	41,273	N/A[2]
Diagnosis	RDTs procured	1,004,875	2,082,600	2,110,000	6,153,350	11,350,825 (8,239,825 distributed)
	Health workers trained in malaria laboratory diagnosis	-	1,370	1,663	2,856	N/A[2]

[1] The numbers reported in this table are up-to-date as of January 1, 2010, and include all 15 PMI focus countries. In addition, during 2009, the USG provided support for case management activities in the Democratic Republic of the Congo, Nigeria, and Sudan; more than 3,000 health workers were trained in the use of ACTs and more than 6.2 million ACTs were procured, of which 5.4 million were distributed. For data by country, see Appendix 2.

[2] A cumulative count of individual health workers trained for Years 1 through 4 of PMI is not provided since some health workers have been trained on more than one occasion.

As control measures in many sub-Saharan African countries have been scaled up, the burden of malaria has been reduced, and an increasing proportion of febrile illnesses are no longer caused by malaria. Therefore, giving malaria treatment based solely on the presence of fever is no longer an acceptable practice, unless diagnostic testing is inaccessible. As countries implement diagnostic testing for malaria, responding to WHO's updated guidance, they are observing a reduction in the percentage of people with fever who receive treatment for malaria because febrile patients without malaria are being screened out, therefore, the ACT coverage indicator related to children under five with a fever no longer accurately reflects progress toward ACT scale-up.

The scale-up of ACTs across the 15 PMI focus countries has progressed rapidly in the last two to three years. To track the availability of ACTs, PMI supported sub-national End-Use Verification surveys in six countries (Ethiopia, Ghana, Kenya, Malawi, Tanzania, and Zambia) during 2009. In Tanzania, PMI's monitoring of ACT stocks in 80 facilities with the End-Use tool found that an average of 93 percent of public health facilities had at least one presentation of an ACT in stock and were able to treat patients. in the other five countries.

Health Systems Strengthening

Improving case management of malaria in African countries presents numerous challenges due to weak health systems. Health worker shortages, infrequent and ineffective training and supervision, weak supply chain management systems, and the lack of quality laboratory services greatly limit a country's ability to deliver high-quality services for malaria and other childhood illnesses.

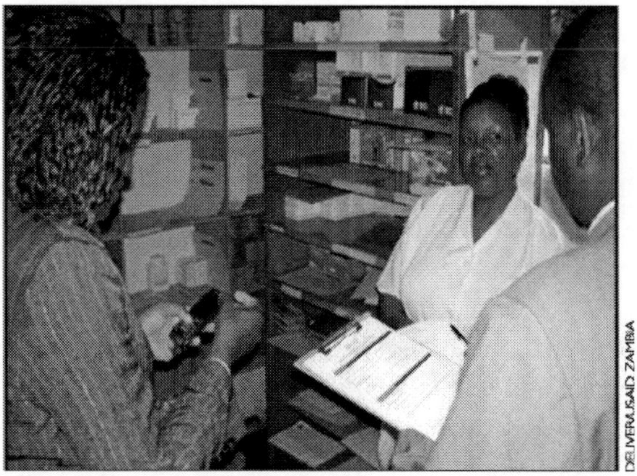

At a health center in Kafue, Zambia, Felistas Mphanza, a Public Health Logistics Officer, collects data on a mobile phone during a PMI End-Use Verification survey, which simplifies and expedites the information gathering process. PMI supported the monitoring of the availability of key malaria commodities through quarterly surveys at health facilities in six PMI focus countries in 2009.

Recognizing these challenges, PMI not only supports procurement and distribution of antimalarial drugs and diagnostic equipment and supplies, but also invests heavily in training and supervision of health workers in malaria laboratory diagnosis and treatment and in strengthening supply chain management systems for essential drugs and supplies. For example, during 2009, PMI provided essential support to the Mozambique Ministry of Health to assist with the implementation of its revised malaria treatment policy (see Voices from the Field on page 34).

Diagnostic Testing for Malaria

Implementation of the new WHO recommendations on diagnostic testing will represent a fundamental change in the management of febrile illnesses and suspected malaria, particularly in sub-Saharan Africa. For more than 50 years, the vast majority of malaria cases have been diagnosed solely on clinical grounds, based on symptoms, and all patients with fevers were presumed to have malaria and were treated accordingly. Microscopic examination of blood films, the gold standard for laboratory diagnosis of malaria, is usually only available at higher-level health Similar results were found facilities. RDTs, which can be used even at the community level by workers with limited training, offer an attractive option to extend diagnostic testing to more peripheral levels.

Although the new WHO guidance related to diagnostic testing of malaria was only recently released, since its launch in 2005, PMI has been supporting the procurement of RDTs; microscopes, and laboratory supplies; refurbishing national malaria reference laboratories; supporting laboratory technician training and supervision; and strengthening quality control programs forlaboratories. During 2009, PMI:

- Provided support to the **Uganda** NMCP to train 1,100 laboratory technicians and clinicians in the performance and appropriate use of malaria microscopy and RDTs. In addition, PMI supported the training of more than 1,350 health workers on malaria case management;

- Procured 1.6 million multispecies RDTs, 57 micro-scopes, and 40 centrifuges for anemia testing for **Ethiopia**, where the diagnosis and treatment of malaria are more complicated than in other countries in sub- Saharan Africa, since infections can be caused by both *P. falciparum* and *P.vivax*;
- Trained 24 district-level laboratory and clinical super-visors in Benin to conduct on-site supervision and training of facility-based laboratory technicians and clinicians in the performance and use of diagnostic testing for malaria. To date, 60 health facilities have received two rounds of supervisory visits. In addition, PMI procured 20 microscopes to replace missing or poorly functioning microscopes in selected health facilities.

Supply Chain Management

Well-functioning supply chain management systems are critical to improving the diagnosis and treatment of malaria. This includes forecasting of drug and diagnostic testing needs, procurement, storage, transportation, inventory management, and rational use of commodities by health workers. Since its launch in 2005, PMI has focused attention on strengthening focus country supply chain management systems. During the past year:

- Following reports of RDT stockouts, PMI supported the MOH in Zambia to conduct a quantification exercise for RDTs in March 2009. As a result of this assessment, the MOH requested assistance with an emergency procurement of more than 2 million RDTs, which were purchased through PMI's Central Emergency Procurement Fund and other funds. However, an updated RDT gap analysis in September indicated that, due to delays in funding from other donors, the country would exhaust its existing supplies of RDTs by February 2010. Again at the request of the MOH, PMI initiated another procurement of nearly 2 million RDTs. This should cover needs for the next seven or eight months when funds from other donors should provide Zambia with adequate supplies of RDTs to last until April 2011.

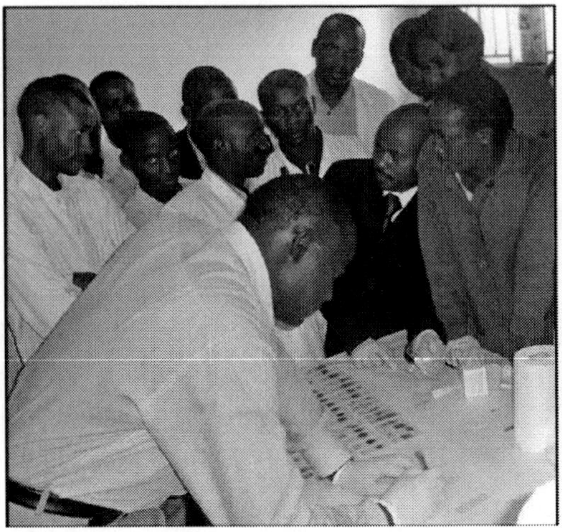

UGANDA MALARIA SURVEILLANCE PROJECT

Participants in a PMI-supported training program in malaria laboratory diagnosis in Uganda review how to make blood smears.

- To avert a nationwide stockout of ACTs in Kenya, PMI procured 7.8 million ACT treatments, of which 6 million were distributed to all 5,000 public health facilities in the country.
- Following an assessment of ACT stocks in the Central Medical Stores in Benin, PMI averted the waste of 600,000 ACT treatments that were at risk of expiring by working with partners to redistribute the drugs to health facilities where they could be used before expiring.

Assuring Quality of Drugs and Diagnostics

PMI procures antimalarial commodities through a rigorous quality assurance/quality control process. For pharmaceuticals, this includes analytic testing to verify product integrity. All drug products are approved by a stringent regulatory authority or through the WHO prequalification program. In April 2009, WHO, CDC, and the Foundation for Innovative New Diagnostics (FIND) published the results of the first round of quality tests on 41 different malaria RDT kits produced by 21 manufacturers. The results of this testing identified a number of test kits that performed very accurately and others that did not perform as well, particularly at low parasite densities. PMI's quality assurance/quality control process for RDTs incorporates the results of the WHO/CDC/FIND Round 1 product testing and also includes preshipment lot testing of all RDTs procured by PMI.

An emerging problem in combating malaria throughout much of the developing world is the sale of counterfeit, adulterated, and poor quality drugs. Not only do these drugs fail to deliver the appropriate treatment to individual patients – putting their lives at risk – but also they contribute to the emergence of drug-resistant strains of malaria.

PMI has supported the Food and Drug Board (FDB) of Ghana to establish a drug quality monitoring program. by working with partners The program trained FDB and NMCP staff on anti-malarial drug sampling and testing, purchased portable drug testing equipment, and provided technical support for the first round of testing. The results showed that out of 447 drug samples screened, 127 (28 percent) failed basic testing. Of the 62 samples subjected to full laboratory testing, 69 percent failed to comply with official standards. Subsequently, following a tip from a consumer, PMI-donated equipment was used to identify counterfeit ACTs. The Ghana FDB moved swiftly to remove the counterfeit products from the market, levied heavy fines, and issued warnings to pharmacies where the products were found. PMI is now working with INTERPOL and the FDB to trace the origin of the counterfeit drugs.

PMI also supported similar postmarketing antimalarial drug quality control assessments in Benin, Ethiopia, Madagascar, Senegal, and Uganda.

Community Case Management of Malaria

In most African countries, more than half of all patients with suspected malaria first seek treatment outside the formal health system. To bring health services to the community level, a variety of community-based approaches are being used. Programs range from training village volunteers to provide treatment for malaria alone to training paid community health workers (CHWs) to manage multiple diseases, including malaria.

Early experiences in many countries, including Senegal, Rwanda, and Madagascar, have demonstrated that both access to and timeliness of malaria treatment can be greatly improved through community-based approaches. Moreover, early evidence from some countries has suggested that community case management increases the number of children with fever who receive treatment within 24 hours of onset of symptoms and reduces the risk of developing severe malaria.

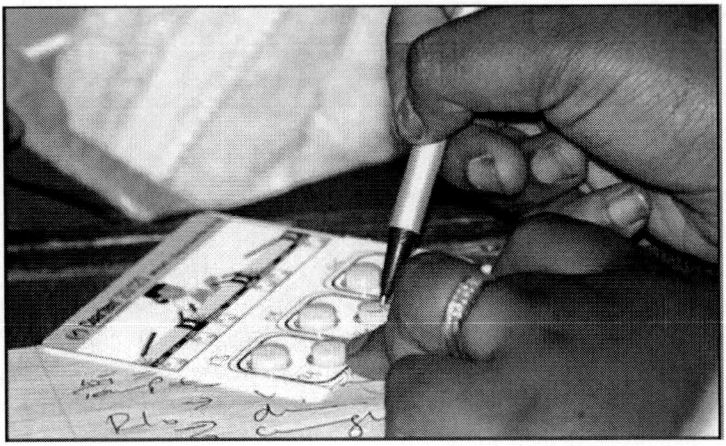

ARTURO SANABRIA/SI

At the Kanyama Urban Health Center in Lusaka, Zambia, a health worker explains how to follow the three-day treatment schedule to ensure that a mother understands how to give this ACT to her child.

PMI support has been essential in Malawi, Rwanda, and Senegal in facilitating the training and supervision of CHWs and developing and maintaining systems to ensure constant supplies of antimalarial drugs and other commodities at the village level. During 2009, PMI:

- Supported expansion of community case management in Rwanda within the context of community integrated management of childhood illness. Eight of the 10 PMI-supported districts have initiated community case management, and a total of 162,000 ACT treatments (procured by Global Fund) were distributed through trained CHWs. In addition, another 233,000 ACT treatments (procured by Global Fund) were distributed to children under the age of five through private sector outlets. Refresher training also was conducted for more than 7,672 health care providers, CHWs, and private sector dispensers;
- Continued to support an integrated community case management program for childhood illness in seven regions in Senegal, which provides treatment of pneumonia, diarrheal disease, and malaria at the community level. PMI also continued to support the community-based treatment of malaria nationwide and worked closely with the NMCP to support the expansion of its home-based management of malaria program, which grew from 21 village volunteers in three districts in 2008 to 408 volunteers in 25 districts at the end of 2009.

This new program targets communities located more than five kilometers from a health facility, where access to health care is particularly difficult. Volunteers selected by their communities are trained in the use of RDTs and treatment with ACTs. Since the program began, 6,200 people have been tested for malaria, of which 2,100 were positive and 2,060 were treated with ACTs. No deaths have been attributed to malaria n these communities since the program began; and

- Procured more than 300,000 ACT treatments to support the scale-up of community case management in Malawi. PMI, with additional USAID maternal and child health funding, also supported the supervision of health surveillance assistants who manage village clinics in eight districts. Additional support was provided for the development of standardized community case management case reporting forms and a logistics management information system to monitor the consumption of drugs at the community level.

PMI also supports community case management through the sale of subsidized ACTs in trained and licensed private sector drug shops:

In Rwanda, PMI has supported the NMCP's strategy of case management for children under five in the private sector by introducing an ACT, branded as PRIMO, into private sector pharmacies and over-the-counter outlets (see photo on page 29). The NMCP has developed a program to register and accredit these marketing and subsidized pricing scheme appropriate treatment of malaria for children under five.

VOICES FROM THE FIELD

PMI-Supported Launch of New Treatment Guidelines in Mozambique

In 2007, the Ministry of Health of Mozambique announced its intention to adopt artemether-lumefantrine (AL) as the first-line treatment for uncomplicated malaria. From the time of this announcement until the policy was successfully implemented in late 2009, PMI provided support at almost every step, including technical assistance on the development of the new treatment policy and help in developing and printing the materials used to train clinicians in the new treatment policy.

PMI also assisted with forecasting of drug requirements to implement the new policy and procured most of the AL needed for the launch of the policy. In 2009, PMI procured more than 3.5 million ACT treatments for Mozambique. When it was determined that the new malaria treatment would not fit in the current drug kits provided to frontline health facilities, PMI provided the human resources, supplies, and technical assistance to the Central Medical Stores to assemble new malaria drug kits, so they could be delivered in tandem with the other drug kits.

Finally, PMI provided logistical support to provincial and district health authorities to support the cascade training of clinical staff in the new malaria treatment policy. With PMI's support, more than 16,000 health workers were trained in case management with ACTs during 2009. With the full implementation of the new treatment policy, PMI will continue to provide technical and logistical support to all levels of the health system to strengthen supervision of clinical staff and ensure that the new policy is being implemented appropriately.

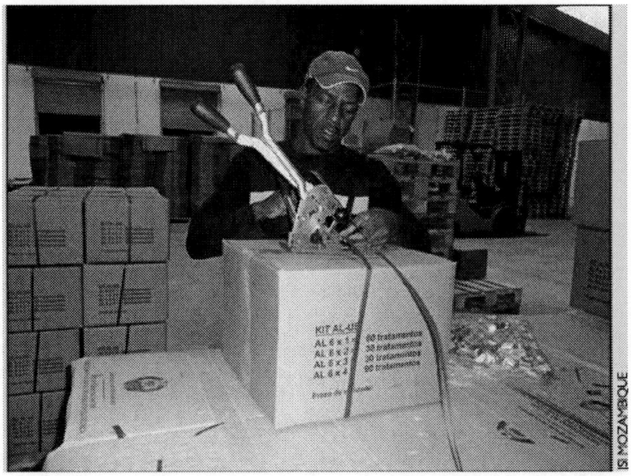

A worker in the Central Medical Stores in Maputo, Mozambique, seals a drug kit containing artemether-lumefantrine, the new first-line treatment of uncomplicated malaria, for use at health facilities and by community health workers.

In Tanzania, PMI supports the sale of subsidized ACTs through private sector Accredited Drug Dispensing Outlets (ADDO). The ADDO program, which included development of policies; standards; trainings; and regulatory systems, transforms unli-censed drug vendors into outlets licensed to dispense ACTs along with other specified prescription drugs.

Future Directions

Despite problems with weak health systems in the 15 PMI focus countries, significant progress has been made in improving malaria diagnosis and treatment.

Continued efforts will be needed, however, to ensure that countries have the capacity to forecast drug requirements, manage stocks, transport drugs and related commodities shops and a to the periphery, and monitor and report consumption.

PMI efforts already have helped lay the groundwork for rapid scale-up of malaria diagnostic testing at health facilities and, in some cases, at the community level in line with new WHO guidelines. Beyond the procurement of RDTs, microscopes, and laboratory supplies, PMI is assisting MOHs to develop appropriate policies and training materials, supporting training and supervision of laboratory and clinical staff in the performance of diagnostic tests, and deploying quality assurance systems for malaria diagnosis.

For more information, please visit the diagnosis and treatment section of the PMI website at

http://www.pmi.gov/technical/acts/index.html.

5. Health Systems, Integration, and Country Capacity

"We must invest in health systems to ensure that all nations have the infrastructure they need to help their citizensthrive. Improving health systems globally creates virtuous cycles: The doctors and nurses who can beat back thescourge of malaria will also be better equipped to combat TB, HIV/AIDS, pneumonia, and other deadly diseases.We must not just help deliver doses; we must help build systems."

– U.S. Ambassador to the United Nations Susan E. Rice, Keynote Address to the U.N. on World Malaria Day, April 24, 2009

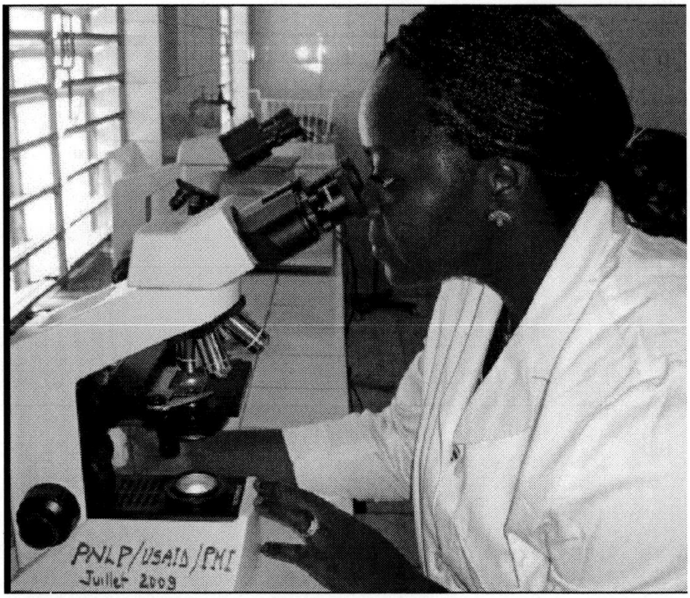

Evelyne Araye, a laboratory technician at the Kouandé Zonal Hospital in Benin, examines a slide under a microscope providedby PMI. Diagnostic testing for malaria enables health care workers to distinguish malaria from other causes of fever.

From the beginning of the President's Malaria Initiative, the USG has coordinated its efforts to scale up life-saving interventions with the need to strengthen health systems capacities of national programs.

Rather than trying to deal simultaneously with all the problems related to health systems in focus countries, PMI has concentrated on a smaller number of areas that present major bottlenecks to scaling up malaria and other critical maternal and child health interventions. These include:

- Supporting pharmaceutical and supply chain management;
- Improving the quality of diagnostic testing;
- Integrating malaria activities within maternal and child health services;
- Building capacities of national malaria control programs;
- Strengthening monitoring and evaluation systems;
- Supporting policy change.

Supporting Pharmaceutical and Supply Chain Management

Weak supply chain management systems have proven to be a significant obstacle to scaling up malaria control efforts in sub-Saharan Africa. In most countries in the region, the capacity to forecast accurately and quantify commodity needs and procure, store, transport, and maintain inventories of commodities is limited. This has resulted in vulnerable supply chains prone to uneven stockouts, expired drugs, and thefts. A direct outcome of these weak supply chains is reduced quality antimalarial drugs as well as other essential maternal and child health medical products. Since it was launched in 2005, PMI has placed a high priority on trying to address these weaknesses. During FY 2009, PMI programmed nearly $9 million for pharmaceutical management activities.

One example of PMI's work in pharmaceutical management in 2009 was an assessment of **Benin's** Central Medical Stores (CAME), which identified serious short comings at all levels of the supply chain management system and found that more than 600,000 ACT treatments in CAME's warehouses were at risk of expiring. interventions with the The assessment revealed weaknesses in the legal status, and build the governance, and internal management of CAME that limited its ability to procure and distribute commodities. Following the assessment, PMI worked with its partners to redistribute the ACTs to health facilities to avoid their expiration. PMI also took the lead in coordinating with other donors to help implement all key recommendations of the assessment. A new drug regulatory framework was developed through consultations with the MOH, CAME's Executive Committee, and other stakeholders, helping to ensure the effectiveness of CAME and a stronger logistics system for all critical drugs.

Improving the Quality of Diagnostic Testing

Accurate diagnosis of what causes fevers is critical not only for clinicians to treat their patients appropriately, but also because it allows NMCPs to accurately monitor the progress of their malaria control efforts. PMI has invested in improving the quality of diagnostic testing for malaria by by microscopy and rapid diagnostic tests in the 15 focus countries. This has included support for training in test methodologies, quality assurance, and quality control systems. These efforts have had the additional benefit of strengthening laboratory diagnostic capabilities more broadly in each country.

At the country level, PMI has worked with national malaria control programs to conduct assessments of focus countries' malaria laboratory diagnostic capabilities. Based on these assessments and in coordination with other partners, such as the U.S. President's Emergency distribution, periodic Plan for AIDS Relief (PEPFAR), PMI attempts to fill gaps by procuring microscopes, microscopy supplies, and access by patients to RDTs. Comprehensive supervision and quality control systems for laboratory technicians are now being implemented in seven PMI countries. In 2009, PMI supported the training of more than 2,800 laboratory staff in the performance of malaria microscopy and RDTs.

PMI also supports refresher training of senior laboratory technicians, pre-service and in-service training of laboratory staff at the health facility level, and establishment of quality control systems. For example, in **Uganda** in 2009, PMI supported the development of a three-day malaria case management training course that can be conducted at the health facility level so as not to disrupt the provision of services. More than 1,300 health workers were trained through these courses. In addition, 1,100 clinical workers and microscopists attended joint diagnostic training classes to promote teamwork and increase clinicians' confidence in test results so that they do not treat patients who have negative malaria test results with ACTs.

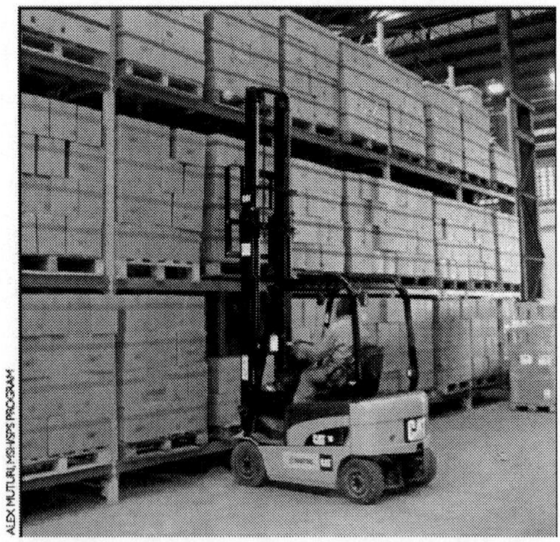

A worker stacks boxes of ACTs in a Medical Supplies Agency warehouse in Embakasi, Kenya. PMI works with national governments to strengthen their drug supply logistics systems.

Integrating Malaria Activities within Maternal and Child Health Services

Malaria prevention and control are key components of integrated maternal and child health programs in Africa. PMI has consistently targeted pregnant women and children under five years of age in its support of malaria prevention and treatment activities, building on existing antenatal and child health services platforms. This approach strengthens health systems in ways that benefit more general maternal and child health programs. During 2009, PMI supported a variety of integrated programs:

- **Community case management of childhood illnesses:** In most African countries, a significant proportion of children with fever or diarrhea are first seen by care- givers who operate outside of the formal health system. To overcome the problems with limited access to facility-based care, many countries are introducing community-based case management of sick children. PMI supports community case management of child-hood illnesses in many of its countries. For example, during 2009, PMI supported training and supervision of community health workers to provide an integrated package of health services and strengthened supply chain management down to the village level in Malawi, Rwanda, and Senegal. In Benin, with co-financing from USAID Maternal and Child Health funds, PMI supported the start-up of a three-year community case management program that provides an integrated package of services, including community-based ACT distribution, treatment of diarrheal disease, health education on immunization, and management of acute respiratory infection for children under five years of age.
- **Focused antenatal care (FANC) services:** PMI supports activities to prevent and treat malaria in pregnancy within the context of broader reproductive health services across the 15 focus countries. Nearly all PMI countries are implementing focused antenatal care of women during their pregnancy and the post- partum period. The objective of FANC is to ensure that antenatal care visits include health promotion and disease prevention activities, early detection and treat- ment of the complications of pregnancy and diseases, birth preparedness, and complication readiness.

- PMI has supported the scale-up of these services in many countries, in several cases in partnership with PEPFAR, by funding pre-service and in-service training of health workers, supportive supervision, job aids, and improved supply chain management of key commodities.

For example, since it began work in Tanzania, PMI has worked to strengthen malaria in pregnancy programs with both Mainland Tanzania's and Zanzibar's Ministries of Health. To increase the uptake of intermittent preventive treatment for pregnant women (IPTp), PMI has focused on improving the quality of antenatal care services through FANC, regular supervision, and at the district level, strengthened supply chain management for critical commodities, such as sulfadoxine-pyrimethamine (SP) for IPTp, insecticide- treated nets (ITNs), and iron. A major thrust of the program is to ensure that all antenatal clinics have at least one provider trained in FANC, and that all districts have ongoing supportive supervision. With PMI support, at least four FANC trainers were trained in each of the 133 districts on the Mainland, and 24 were trained on Zanzibar. These trainers have now trained other health workers, and by the end of 2009, more than 2,000 health providers were trained in total. As a result, more than 60 percent of antenatal care facilities on the Mainland and 67 percent on Zanzibar now have FANC-trained providers.

- **Integrating ITN distribution into maternal and child health services:** Increasing demand for health services and attendance at health facilities benefits all health programs. Since 2000, ITNs have become highly prized commodities throughout Africa. PMI uses the free distribution of ITNs through antenatal and child immunization clinics to attract greater numbers of patients to those clinics. Incorporating free ITN distribution in immunization and other child health campaigns, as PMI has done in Senegal and Angola, also promotes increased participation in those campaigns. In this way, PMI builds upon the investments that the U.S. Government and other development partners are making in the health sector.

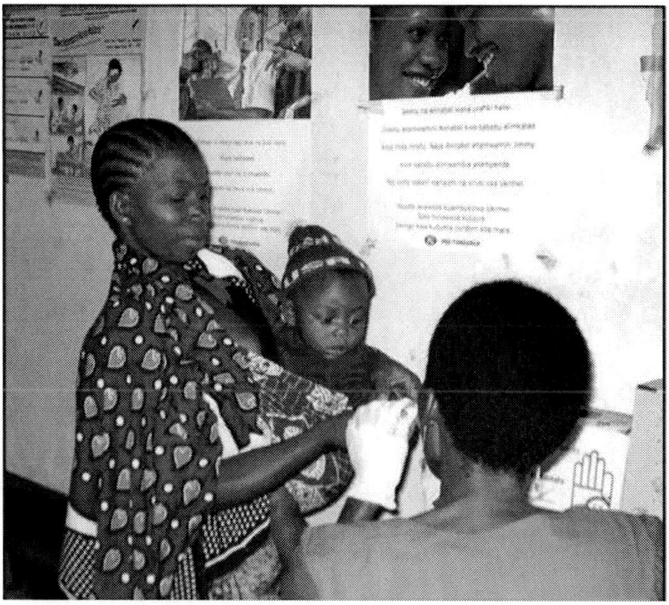

Issa Abrahim holds her son while he has his finger pricked for a rapid diagnostic test for malaria at the Ikwiriri Health Center in Tanzania. Accurate diagnosis of fevers is important for the health of children, for the appropriate use of antimalarial drugs, and for monitoring trends in malaria cases.

Building Capacities of National Malaria Control Programs

PMI's goal is to enable focus country governments to be able to control malaria on their own. Ministries of health (MOHs) and national malaria control programs (NMCPs) must be able to provide leadership combined with technical and managerial skills to plan, implement, evaluate, and adjust, as necessary, their malaria control efforts. Effective NMCPs require staff with expertise in a variety of fields, including entomology, epidemiology, case management, monitoring and evaluation, laboratory diagnosis, supply chain management, behavior change communications, and financial management. During 2009, PMI provided technical assistance to NMCPs in a variety of ways:

- In Benin, PMI promoted an organizational audit of the NMCP that will be used to restructure the program and develop a capacity-building strategy. In order to improve technical capacity, PMI trained

NMCP staff in communications, entomology and epidemiology, and supportive supervision;

- In **Mozambique**, the vector control specialist leading PMI's IRS activities in-country trained 22 NMCP personnel in field entomologic techniques, such as mosquito collections, identification, and insecticide resistance testing, to build local capacity for future vector control activities;
- PMI has worked closely with the **Senegal** NMCP to support development of a quality assurance/quality control (QA/QC) system for laboratory diagnosis. During the last half of 2009, PMI partners trained a total of 86 staff from 11 regions on QA/QC; and
- In **Uganda**, PMI worked with the NMCP to pilot an ITN distribution campaign in three eastern districts ahead of a large-scale distribution in 2010. With support from PMI and other partners, Uganda plans to distribute approximately 17 million ITNs, funded by the Global Fund, by the end of 2010.

Strengthening Monitoring and Evaluation Systems

National malaria control programs must have the capacity to monitor and evaluate their progress, to identify problems in program implementation and allow modifications to be made, and to confirm that those modifications are having their desired effect. PMI works with other partners to help improve the evidence base used by NMCPs, PMI, and other partners to demonstrate progress against malaria. PMI provides support for the development of national monitoring and evaluation (M&E) plans and strategies, national surveys, and the improvement of national health information services. For example, during 2009, PMI:

- Assisted the Rwandan NMCP in updating its National Malaria M&E Strategy and National Strategic Plan for the Prevention and Control of Malaria, and supported a training course on applied M&E for malaria control;
- Worked with NMCPs, the World Health Organization (WHO), and UNICEF to produce the first National Malaria M&E Plan for Ghana and Tanzania;

- Collaborated with the MOH, NMCP, WHO, and other partners to harmonize the collection and reporting of malaria indicators in Ghana; and
- Provided technical guidance to the Zanzibar Malaria Control Program in its efforts to collect and interpret data from the Zanzibar Malaria Early Epidemic Detection System and to publish and disseminate periodic reports.

Supporting Policy Change

In order to maximize the effectiveness of malaria investments, countries must have policies in place that are conducive to effective malaria control. Ministries of health and NMCPs must also develop policies around cross-cutting systems, such as pharmaceutical management, monitoring and evaluation, integrated surveillance, and behavior change communication.

Through its in-country staff and implementing partners, PMI provides technical assistance to MOHs and NMCPs to promote the establishment of sound malaria prevention and treatment policies that reflect internationally accepted best practices. During 2009, PMI:

- Worked with the Ghanaian NMCP and its partners to update guidelines for malaria case management and preventing malaria in pregnancy and assisted in revising training manuals, essential medication lists, and insurance formularies;

- Encouraged the Government of Mali to increase the visibility of the NMCP by raising it to the directorate level within the MOH in 2008 and worked to increase government funding for malaria control to more than $9 million in FY 2009 from about $1 million in FY 2007; and

- Worked with Senegal's NMCP to enact a change in the Ministry of Health's ACT policy that resulted in a declaration that starting on May 1, 2010, ACTs will be provided free of charge in all government health facilities nationwide.

VOICES FROM THE FIELD

Malaria Entomology Revitalized in Zambia

A successful vector control program needs to do more than just spray houses and distribute mosquito nets. It must also have the ability to monitor mosquito populations and their response to vector control measures. The field of malaria entomology was in decline in Zambia for many years, but it attracted renewed interest owing to increased investment in malaria control efforts and interest in malaria elimination. The Ministry of Health, with support from PMI and others, is building entomologic capability to support vector control measures. "In former times, we had entomology technicians in the district who carried out local surveys," reminisces Dr. Cecilia Shinondo, Senior Entomologist and Malaria Specialist for the PMI-supported Health Systems Strengthening Project.

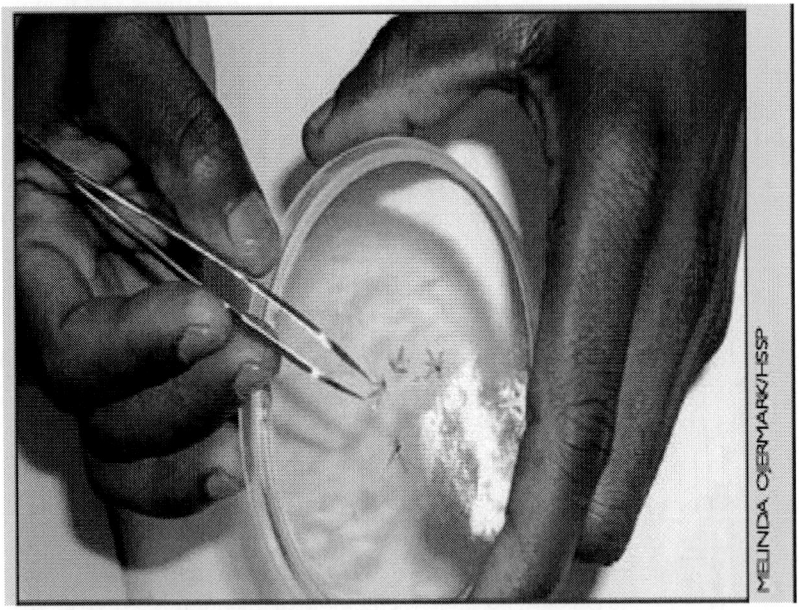

Mosquitoes readied for dissection.

"Today these categories of staff have virtually disappeared, but we are rebuilding capacity in entomology by training university students and district environmental health staff."

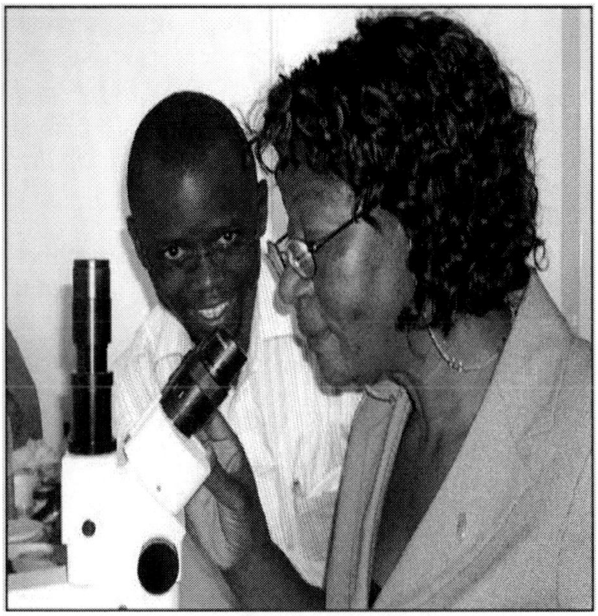

Dr. Cecilia Shinondo, assisted by insectary technician Idan Emmanuel Chabu, identifies mosquito species under a microscope.

The National Malaria Control Center's insectary for rearing mosquitoes was recently refurbished with support from PMI. The insectary's small laboratory is now a center of activity, where students learn to identify and analyze mosquitoes (including dissections) to determine if they carry malaria parasites and changes in population survivorship to monitor the effectiveness of vector control programs. In the adjoining room, a tropical atmosphere prevails. Heaters whirr, and a humidifier emits a steamy vapor. Small mesh cages filled with live adult mosquitoes line the shelves, and water-filled dishes in orderly rows contain larvae and pupae. The goal is to establish a colony of mosquitoes that will be used for training and to monitor the quality and duration of insecticides used in IRS and for ITNs and as a control group for insecticide resistance studies routinely conducted before and after the IRS programs. The painstaking work is paying off, and soon the insectary will have sufficient stock to support training and quality control monitoring for Zambia's vector control programs.

6. PARTNERSHIPS

"While much remains to be done, the tremendous increase in funding for malaria control is resulting in therapid scale-up of today's control tools. This, in turn, is having a profound effect on health – especially the healthof children in sub-Saharan Africa. In a nutshell, development aid for health is working."

– Dr. Margaret Chan, World Health Organization Director-General, December 15, 2009

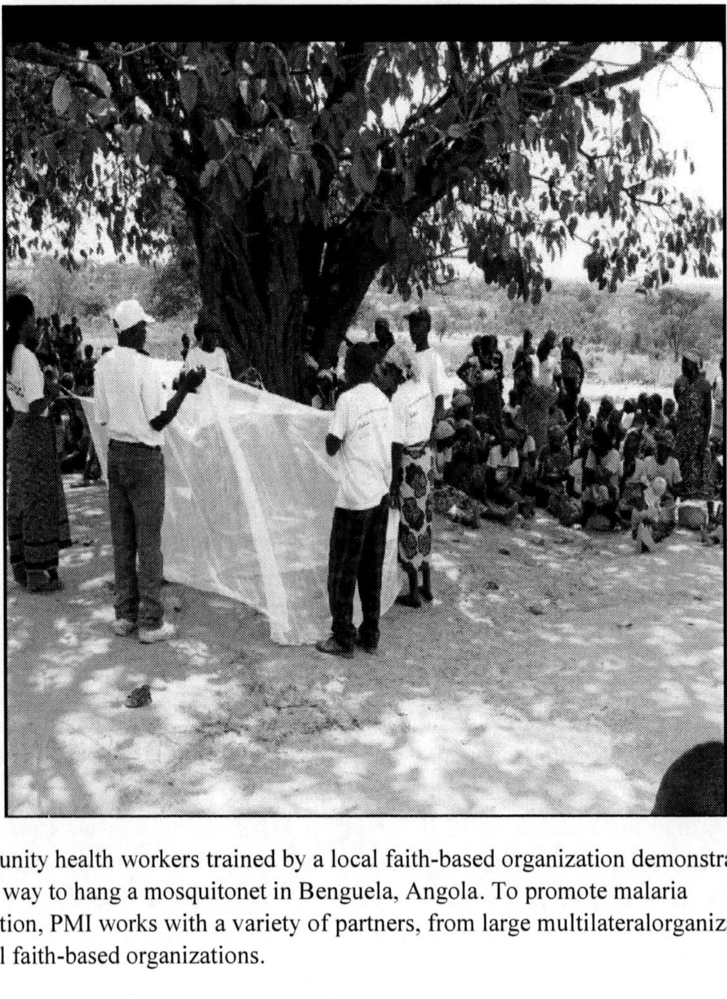

Community health workers trained by a local faith-based organization demonstrate the proper way to hang a mosquitonet in Benguela, Angola. To promote malaria prevention, PMI works with a variety of partners, from large multilateralorganizations to local faith-based organizations.

Progress in scaling up coverage of malaria prevention and treatment interventions depends on effective partnerships. PMI works closely with host country governments; other U.S. Government agencies; international organizations; bilateral, multilateral, and private donors; local and international nongovernmental organizations and faith-based organizations (NGOs and FBOs); and the private sector to ensure that efforts are complementary and support national malaria control strategies and plans.

Multilateral Organizations

As PMI works with NMCPs and in-country partners to sustainably reduce the burden of malaria in Africa, the Initiative also attempts to identify and fill gaps in funding and support from other partners. In the 15 focus countries, PMI also coordinates its efforts with the multilateral and bilateral institutions and private sector organizations (see Table, below). PMI sits on the Board of Directors of the Roll Back Malaria (RBM) Partnership and is an active member of the U.S. Government's delegation to The Global Fund. During 2009, PMI:

- Worked in Kenya with its pharmaceutical management partners, including the Division of Malaria Control, Kenya Medical Supply Agency, and the Global Fund Procurement and Supply Chain Consortium, to monitor stocks of the first-line antimalarial drug, an artemisinin-based combination therapy (ACT). When an impending ACT stockout was identified, PMI made an emergency procurement of 7.8 million ACT treatments, of which 6 million were distributed to all 5,000 public health facilities nationwide;
- Contributed nearly $1 million in financial support to a UNICEF-led nationwide disease prevention campaign in Angola, which included routine vaccination, deworming, vitamin A administration, and the distribution of 1.8 million free ITNs to pregnant women and children under the age of one;
- Supported the launch of the 2009–2010 mass long-lasting ITN distribution campaign in Madagascar in collaboration with UNICEF, the principal recipient of the Global Fund malaria grant (PSI), the International Federation of Red Cross and Red Crescent Societies, the Malagasy Red Cross, WHO, and the NMCP (see Voices from the Field on page 16).

- Facilitated the creation of a technical working group in Benin to coordinate, plan, and oversee the quantification and procurement of malaria commodities at the national level. The working group is hosted by the Ministry of Health and includes all major donors supporting malaria activities in Benin: the principal recipients of the Global Fund (Catholic Relief Services and Africare), UNICEF, the World Bank Booster Program, the African Development Bank Malaria Support Project, and PMI implementing partners;
- Played an active role in all RBM working groups, including the Monitoring and Evaluation Reference Group, where PMI collaborates with partners to develop guidelines on malaria indicators and measurement tools and on the timing and funding of malaria surveys; and

Examples of PMI Partners in Malaria Control.

Multilateral and Bilateral Partners	Private Sector and Foundations
• Roll Back Malaria Partnership • United Nations Secretary-General's Special Envoy for Malaria • World Health Organization • United Nations Children's Fund (UNICEF) • The Global Fund to Fight AIDS, Tuberculosis and Malaria (Global Fund) • World Bank • United Kingdom Department for International Development	• Malaria No More • Global Business Coalition • Bill and Melinda Gates Foundation • United Nations Foundation (Nothing but Nets) • ExxonMobil Foundation • Clinton Foundation • Carter Center

- Continued to provide technical support to African countries through the RBM Harmonization Working Group in the preparation of their Global Fund malaria grant applications. In Rounds 7 through 9, the success rate of malaria proposals that received technical support from the Working Group increased to between 54 and 78 percent from 32 percent in Round 6.

Interagency Partnerships

PMI recognizes the importance of taking a government- wide approach to foreign assistance. During 2009, the Initiative continued to coordinate activities and work with other USG agencies and programs in focus countries, including the Peace Corps, the Department of Defense, the U.S. President's Emergency Plan for AIDS Relief (PEPFAR), and others.

During 2009, Peace Corps volunteers in Senegal, working with PMI, organized and led the distribution of more than 20,000 ITNs in the communities where the volunteers live and work. In addition, they helped with a universal ITN coverage campaign in two of the health districts with the highest prevalence of malaria.

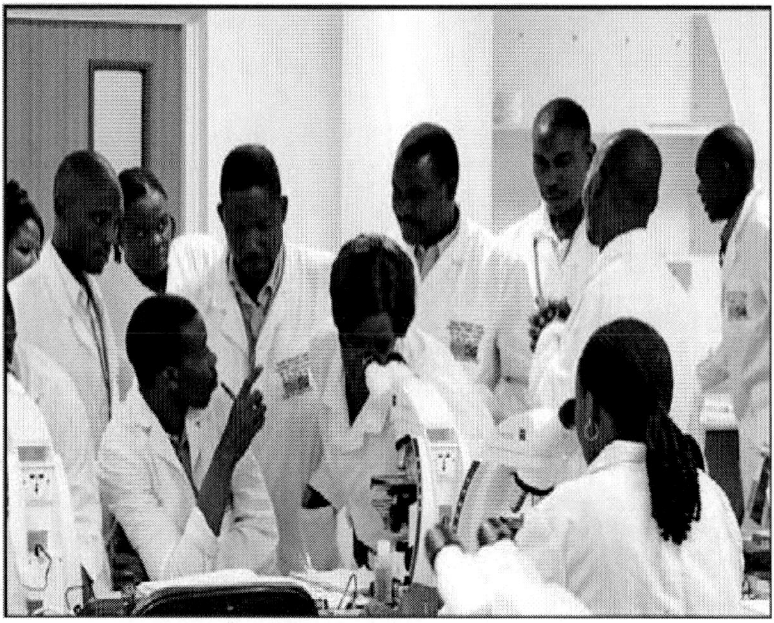

MAJ. ERIC WAGAR, KEMRI/USAMRU-KENYA

Tanzanian medical laboratory technicians receive malaria microscopy training during a workshop led by a team of U.S. Army instructors from the U.S. Army Medical Research Unit and the Combined Joint Task Force for the Horn of Africa.

PMI collaborated with a team of U.S. Army instructors from the Combined Joint Task Force for the Horn of Africa and the U.S. Army Medical Research Unit in Kenya to provide malaria microscopy training to 20

Tanzanian medical laboratory technicians. The training took place at the Ministry of Health's new National Health Laboratory and Quality Assurance Training Center in Tanzania's capital, Dar es Salaam, which had recently been renovated and equipped with PEPFAR funding.

The U.S. Department of Defense has also provided two U.S. Navy entomologists, detailed through CDC, to support PMI operations in Ghana, Malawi, and Mali. Staff from the Armed Forces Pest Management Board also helped develop integrated vector management materials for PMI focus countries.

PMI and PEPFAR have 10 focus countries in common (Angola, Ethiopia, Ghana, Kenya, Malawi, Mozambique, Rwanda, Tanzania, Uganda, and Zambia). Since both programs target pregnant women, there are programmatic reasons to combine intermittent preventive treatment for pregnant women (IPTp) and the distribution of insecticide-treated nets (ITNs) with services for the prevention of mother-to-child transmission of HIV (PMTCT). During 2009, PMI-PEPFAR collaborations included the following:

- In Ethiopia, PMI and PEPFAR worked together to develop behavior change communication (BCC) activities to increase prevention and treatment of malaria, improve antenatal clinic attendance, and strengthen PMTCT.
- In Uganda, PMI and PEPFAR worked with 11 large businesses to improve access to and usage of a broad range of health services among company employees, their dependents, and the surrounding communities. PMI support included the provision of nearly 46,000 IPTp treatments and 100,000 free ITNs to pregnant women.

Private Sector Partners

During 2009, PMI continued to build on its partnerships with the private sector:

- In Angola, for the third consecutive year, the ExxonMobil Foundation made a $1 million donation to supplement PMI support for national and international NGOs to help scale up ACTs, ITNs, and IPTp in nine of Angola's 18 provinces where access to health services is limited. As a result, 4,150 health workers were trained on various aspects of malaria treatment or prevention, including pharmaceutical management, diagnosis and treatment with ACTs, distribution of ITNs, and behavior change communication. These trainings were followed up with more than 1,500 supervisory visits to health facilities.

- In Ghana, PMI's indoor residual spraying (IRS) activities have benefited from the experience of the private mining company, AngloGold Ashanti, which has been conducting IRS in Obuasi District since 2005 (see Voices from the Field on page 22).
- In Zambia, the Mopane and Konkola Copper Mines and the Zambia Sugar Company coordinates IRS activities with PMI and the NMCP.
- In Benin, PMI has supported the NMCP to develop a framework to distribute donor-funded malaria commodities to private health clinics. The framework includes a plan for progressive scale-up beginning with faith-based clinics, private socially franchised clinics, and clinics affiliated with the International Planned Parenthood Federation. Previously, donor-supplied commodities were only distributed to public health facilities, although it is estimated that more than 50 percent of the population seek care from private health facilities. Since October 2009, the NMCP has started to involve these private clinics in the distribution of ITNs, drugs for IPTp, ACTs, and microscopes.
- In Rwanda and Tanzania, PMI supported the NMCPs' policy of community case management through the sale of subsidized ACTs in trained and licensed private sector drug shops.

Nongovernmental Organizations

In many African countries, NGOs, FBOs, and community-based organizations have strong bases of operations in underserved, rural areas where malaria is a major public health problem and formal health services are limited. Through support to these groups, PMI helps build local capacity and program sustainability and improves access to critical malaria prevention and treatment services at the community level. Due to their close contact with local residents, these organizations can facilitate behavior change communication activities to help families prevent and treat malaria. To date, PMI has supported nearly 200 nonprofit organizations; more than 45 of these are FBOs. For example, during 2009, PMI:

Amazon and Mekong Regional Initiatives

In addition to funding malaria activities in sub-Saharan Africa, USAID supports regional malaria programs in Latin America through the Amazon Malaria Initiative (Bolivia, Brazil, Colombia, Ecuador, Guyana, Peru, and Suriname) and in Southeast Asia through the Mekong Malaria Programme (Burma, Cambodia, Lao PDR, Thailand, Vietnam, and Yunnan Province, China).

USAID support for the Mekong Malaria Programme in FY 2009 was $6.5 million. Working with WHO, Global Fund, the Bill and Melinda Gates Foundation, national malaria control programs, NGOs, the private sector, and with technical assistance from the CDC, the program has established a network of drug resistance and drug quality monitoring sites, provided support for pharmaceutical management and for a common monitoring and evaluation framework throughout the Mekong region. Artemisinin-resistant *falciparum* malaria was first detected in western Cambodia, and decreased sensitivity to artemisinin has now been found in several other sites in the region. The Malaria Programme has supported behavior change efforts related to malaria prevention and treatment for migrant populations, community-based malaria activities in western Cambodia, and development of a model for malaria elimination in Thailand.

USAID FY 2009 support for the Amazon Malaria Initiative was $5 million. Working with the Pan American Health Organization, ministries of health, and national research organizations, between 2000 and 2007, the Initiative helped all countries in the Amazon Basin change their national malaria treatment policies to ACTs and then to implement those new policies. This change in first-line drugs for the treatment of malaria is believed to have contributed to the one-third reduction in the number of malaria cases reported in the region over the same period, as well as a drop in the numbers of cases of the more severe *falciparum* malaria. In collaboration with its partners, USAID also supported technical assistance to improve pharma-ceutical management, strengthen national drug quality control laboratories, pilot studies on the use of rapid diagnostic tests for malaria, and establish systems for monitoring insecticide resistance in mosquitoes.

- Supported Senegal's NMCP to hold its first nationwide distribution of nearly 2.3 million free long-lasting ITNs to children under five in June and October 2009. This campaign involved nearly 20 different local and international organizations, including local and international NGOs, United Nations agencies, two different Red Cross affiliates, a manufacturer of long-lasting ITNs, and a World Bank-funded project. PMI contributed 380,000 nets and about 30 percent of the total operational costs. Advocacy by PMI attracted an additional 86,000 nets from the Canadian Red Cross, the Against Malaria Foundation, and the Sumitomo Chemical Company, as well as support for operations from World Vision and ChildFund Senegal; and
- Partnered with local NGOs and FBOs to continue humanitarian services when the political crisis led to USG restrictions that prohibited direct support to the Government of Madagascar. During Madagascar's ITN mass distribution campaign, PMI supported two local FBOs to deliver 1 million long-lasting ITNs at the community level. PMI also partnered with and supported the Malagasy Red Cross to conduct indoor residual spraying in six health districts, protecting more than 1,270,000 people.

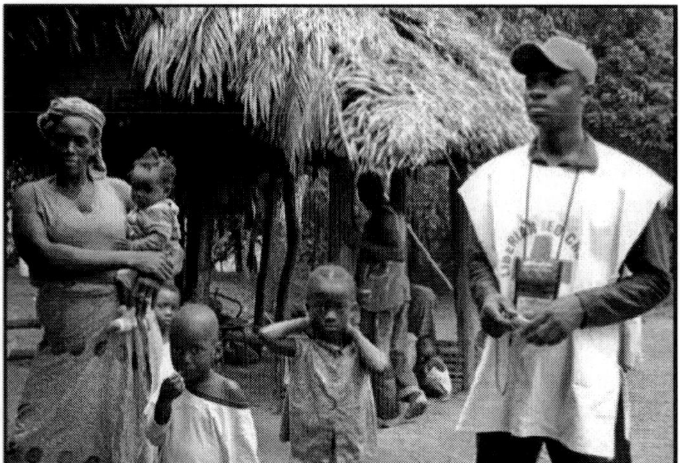

CANADIAN RED CROSS

In Liberia, non-governmental organizations, such as the Red Cross, provide significant support to the MOH to ensure the provision of health services in the areas where they work.

Malaria Communities Program

The Malaria Communities Program (MCP) is a $30 million initiative created in December 2006 to support the efforts of communities and indigenous organizations tives of MCP are to identify and support potential new partners and networks of organizations to combat malaria in PMI focus countries. The objectives of MCP are to identify and support potential newpartners and networks of organizations uniquely positioned to work at the community level and increase localcapacity to undertake community-based malaria prevention and treatment activities.

To date, MCP has awarded 20 grants to 18 organizations that are implementing activities in 12 PMI countries; seven new grants were awarded in September 2009. Some examples of MCP-supported activities during FY 2009 include (see also Voices from the Field on page 46):

- *Ajuda de Desenvolvimento de Povo Angola* enlisted nearly 100 school teachers and 3,700 students in a community malaria advocacy network in Zaire Province in northern Angola. This network mobilized communities in three districts to recognize symptoms of malaria, promote health-seeking behaviors, and distribute more than 3,500 long-lasting insecticide- treated mosquito nets.
- Concern Universal, in Malawi, reached approximately 5,000 mothers with messages on the importance of prompt care seeking for suspected malaria; and 2,500 pregnant women with messages on IPTp through health talks and home visits conducted by health surveillance assistants (a cadre of CHWs). In addition, 166,000 people were reached with messages on ITN use during open-air mass information campaigns that were conducted in communities and major trading centers.
- Lutheran World Relief and its partner, the Evangelical Lutheran Church in Tanzania, were able to extend malaria prevention and control activities from five to ten underserved rural dioceses in mainland Tanzania. A total of 160 senior diocesan staff and 330 parish malaria volunteers were trained and were able to reach nearly 377,000 community members and parishioners in 4,180 participation sessions during church services, house-to-house visits, open space evangelism, church choir, confirmation sessions, and diocesan retreat events and meetings. In addition, nearly 58,400 preschool and Sunday

school students were reached with behavior change materials and malaria messages.

VOICES FROM THE FIELD

Collaboration with a Community-Based Organization Is Key to a Successful ITN Distribution Campaign in Liberia

EQUIP Liberia, a Malaria Communities Program grantee, played a major role in the implementation of a free long- lasting ITN distribution campaign in Nimba County, Liberia, conducted in May–June 2009. EQUIP worked closely with PMI, the Nimba County Health Team, the Ministry of Health, and the national malaria control program to conduct the campaign. The long-lasting ITNs for the campaign were procured and transported to the county level by PMI, while EQUIP assisted the County Health Team to oversee the distribution of nets from the county level down to communities.

Over a period of two weeks, 530 community health volunteers trained by EQUIP Liberia distributed more than 180,000 free ITNs in all six districts of Nimba County, often transporting the bales of nets by foot or even canoe when roads were impassable. Volunteers went from house to house to ensure that each household received three nets and to share information about the importance of using a net to prevent malaria. Because ownership of an ITN does not ensure that it is properly used, the volunteers were equipped with nails and cords to help families hang their nets properly.

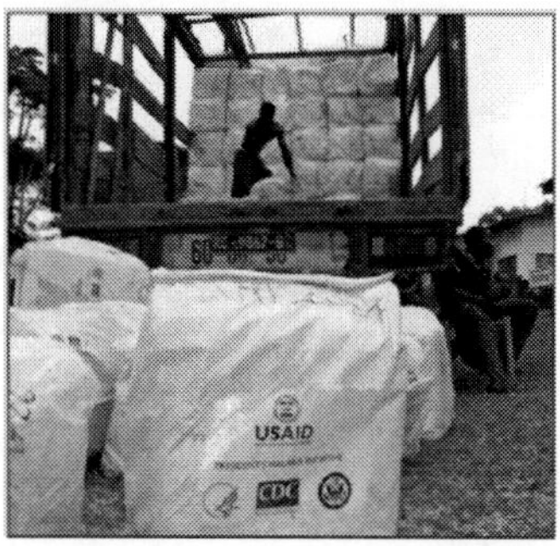

Workers unload bales of insecticide-treated mosquito nets for distribution in Nimba County, Liberia. EQUIP Liberia trained 530 community health volunteers to distribute free ITNs in all six districts.

7. OUTCOMES AND IMPACT

"As we continue to make progress in the fight against malaria, we make important gains toward meeting theMillennium Development Goals related to poverty reduction, child survival, maternal health and reducingmalaria deaths."

– Rear Admiral R.T. Ziemer, USN (ret), U.S. Global Malaria Coordinator, December 15, 2009

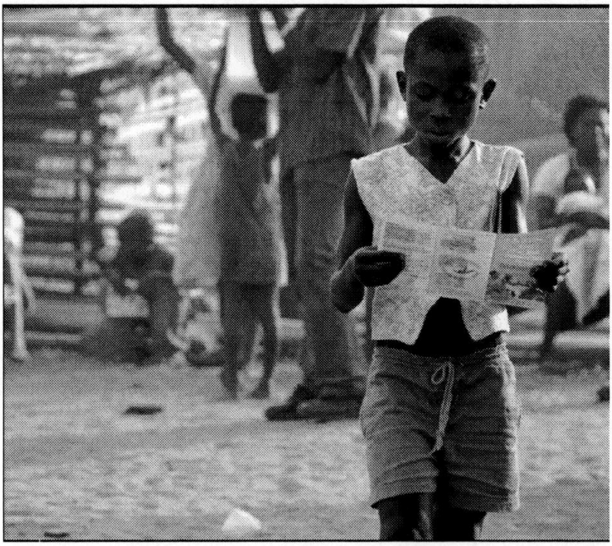

A young Ghanaian girl reads a malaria prevention brochure as she walks through her village. The President's Malaria Initiative isscaling up resources for malaria prevention and treatment to reduce the to burden of malaria and help relieve poverty on theAfrican continent. Information and education are key components of PMI's programs.

The goal of PMI is to reduce malaria-related deaths by 50 percent across the 15 focus countries. This will be achieved by expanding coverage of four highly effective malaria prevention and treatment measures to 85 percent of the most vulnerable populations – pregnant women and children under five years of age. The package of interventions consists of insecticide-treated mosquito nets (ITNs), indoor residual spraying (IRS) with insecticides, intermittent preventive treatment for pregnant women (IPTp), and artemisinin-based combination therapy (ACT).

PMI's Monitoring and Evaluation Strategy

As a member of the global Roll Back Malaria Partnership (RBM), PMI supports efforts to standardize approaches to monitoring and evaluation (M&E) of malaria prevention and treatment measures by national malaria control programs (NMCPs) and their major partners, including The Global Fund to Fight AIDS, Tuberculosis and Malaria (Global Fund), World Bank, World Health Organization (WHO), and UNICEF. PMI's approach to evaluating the impact of malaria control measures is in line with the recommendationsspecific symptoms of malaria, and the lack of laboratory of the RBM Partnership Monitoring and Evaluation Reference Group.

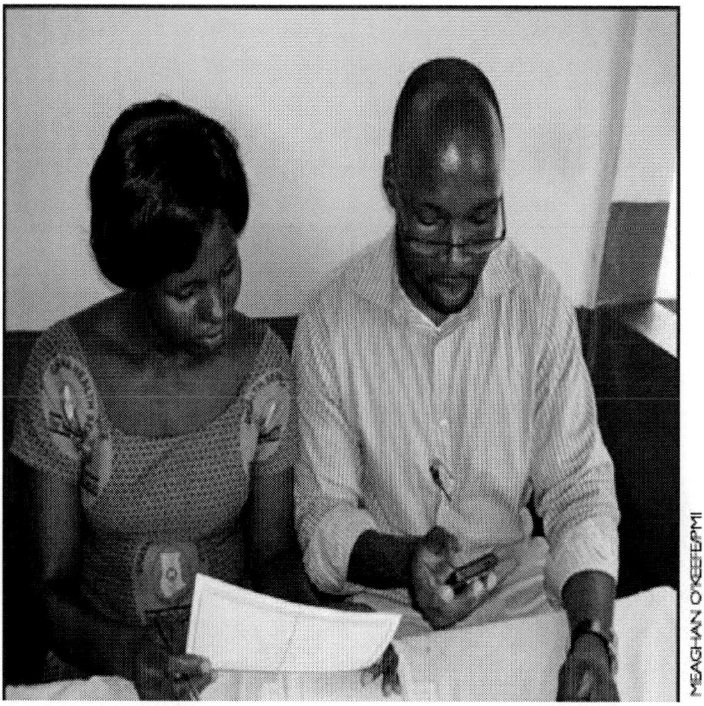

A clinical nurse with the Ghana Health Services reviews case management data with a colleague, who enters the data into a cell phone for analysis. Ongoing monitoring of data is used to improve programs, while periodic evaluations are used to determine whether a program is reaching its goals.

Measuring Impact

PMI defines health impact in two ways:

- Reductions in malaria parasitemia and anemia (which has been shown to be closely associated with malaria infections) among children under five years of age; and
- Reductions in both all-cause and malaria-related mortality in the same population.

Malaria-related mortality is very difficult to measure with any degree of accuracy. Although malaria is responsible for a large proportion of deaths in children under five in sub-Saharan Africa, most of those deaths occur outside health facilities and are not registered, nor is an accurate, specific cause of death assigned. Even within the health system, it may be difficult to determine whether or not malaria was the primary cause of death due to the variety of health problems affecting young children, the non-specific symptoms of malaria, and the lack of laboratory diagnostic capacity in many countries.

Because of these difficulties, PMI is using a multipronged approach recommended by the RBM Monitoring and Evaluation Reference Group to measure change in malaria-related mortality across its 15 focus countries.[1] This consists of monitoring trends in the coverage of malaria control interventions, as well as the multiple factors that could influence childhood mortality, malaria-related morbidity (i.e., parasitemia and anemia), and all-cause mortality in children under five. If reductions in all-cause under-five mortality can be demonstrated along with improvements in the coverage of malaria interventions and reductions in malaria parasitemia and anemia, and no other explanations for these reductions can be identified (such as rainfall, changes in immunization rates, etc.), then it is likely that the reductions in all-cause mortality are due in large part to malaria control efforts. The greater the reductions in all-cause under-five mortality, malaria parasitemia and anemia, and the greater the increases in coverage of malaria control measures, the more likely the association between malaria control activities and reduced malaria-related mortality.

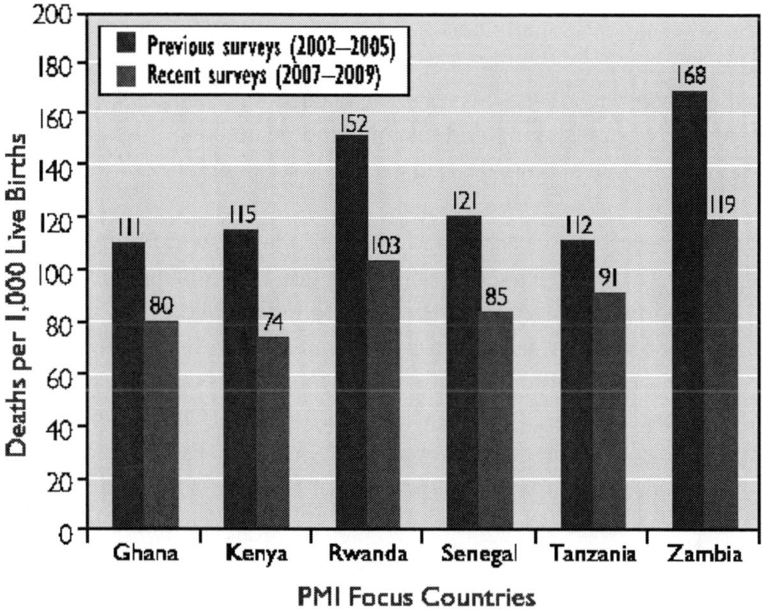

Note: The countries included in this graph are those PMI focus countries for which there are two data points from nationwide household surveys for the indicator.

Figure 1. Reductions in All-Cause Mortality Rates of Children Under Five in Six PMI Countries.

Country-Specific Impact in PMI Focus Countries

The final PMI evaluation of the impact of malaria control efforts across all 15 focus countries will not be completed until early 2012, but there is already evidence that progress is being made. Six of the 15 PMI countries (Ghana, Kenya, Rwanda, Senegal, Tanzania, and Zambia) have had nationwide household surveys conducted in 2002–2005 (during a period when USG funding for malaria control in Africa was rapidly increasing) and again in 2007–20 09. Working with national governments and other donors, PMI and previous USG malaria assistance have helped to scale up rapidly malaria prevention and treatment measures in each of these countries. In all six of these countries, substantial reductions in all-cause mortality in children under five have been documented, ranging from 19 to 36 percent (see Figure 1, above). At the same time, these six countries showed large increases in coverage of malaria prevention and treatment measures and declines in malaria illnesses in outpatient departments and hospitalizations for malariain children under five.

Marked increases in the coverage of malaria interventions, reductions in the prevalence of parasitemia and anemia, and declines in all-cause mortality in children under five are already being seen. For example:

- In Senegal, a 30 percent reduction in all-cause mortality in children under five between 2005 and 2008 has been documented. Although several factors may be involved, it is highly likely that this dramatic reduction is due at least in part to rapid increases in the coverage of malaria interventions. Household ownership of one or more ITNs has increased from 36 percent in 2006 to 60 percent in 2008. The proportion of pregnant women who received two or more doses of IPTp increased from 12 to 52 percent between 2005 and 2008. At the end of 2007, Senegal introduced RDTs for malaria in all of its health facilities, and in 2008, 73 percent of all suspected malaria cases were tested. Although no national-level baseline data are available to compare malaria prevalence, fewer than 6 percent of children under five had malaria parasites in the 2008 nationwide survey, a level much lower than would be expected in most West African countries. USAID has supported malaria control efforts in Senegal since 1999. In FY 2006, $2.2 million in PMI funding was provided, followed by $16.7 million in FY 2007, $15.9 million in FY 2008, and $15.7 million in FY 2009.
- In Zambia, the proportion of households with at least one ITN has increased from 38 percent in 2006 to 62 percent in 2008. More importantly, the use of ITNs by children under five almost doubled from 24 percent in 2006 to 41 percent in 2008. The National Malaria Control Program of Zambia estimates that, since 2003, more than 7 million ITNs have been distributed throughout the country. During the same time period, the prevalence of anemia among children six months to five years of age declined by 71 percent, from 14 to just 4 percent, and malaria parasite prevalence dropped from 22 to 10 percent. It is highly likely that these results contributed significantly to the drop in all-cause under- five mortality from 168 deaths per 1,000 live births in 2002 to 119 per 1,000 in 2007. USAID has supported malaria control efforts in Zambia since 2002, including $7.6 million in FY 2006. PMI provided $9.5 million in FY 2007, followed by $14.9 million in FY 2008, and $14.7 million in FY 2009.

- Analysis of household survey data from Rwanda showed that between 2005 and 2008, ITN use in children under five increased from 13 to 58 percent. Over approximately the same time period, the proportion of hospital deaths attributed to malaria fell from 41 to 16 percent. All-cause mortality in children under five also declined by 32 percent between 2005 and 2008. USAID has supported malaria control efforts in Rwanda since 2002. In FY 2006, PMI provided $1.5 million in funding, followed by $20 million in FY 2007, $16.9 million in FY 2008, and $16.3 million in FY 2009.
- In Tanzania, all-cause under-five mortality fell from 112 deaths per 1,000 live births in 2005 to 91 per 1,000 in 2007. At about the same time, household ownership of ITNs increased from 23 percent in 2005 to 38 percent in 2007. A recent survey showed that children who slept under an ITN in Tanzania were 40 percent less likely to have malaria parasites in their blood than children who did not sleep under an ITN.[2] In the capital, Dar es Salaam, malaria prevalence fell from 24 percent in 2004 to just 4 percent in 2008[3], and the prevalence of severe anemia in children six months to five years of age fell by 30 percent between 2004 and 2007. USAID supported malaria control efforts in Tanzania between 1999 and 2005, including $2 million in FY 2005. Beginning in FY 2006, PMI provided $11.5 million in funding, $31 million in FY 2007, $33.7 million in FY 2008, and $35 million in FY 2009.
- Kenya experienced a substantial reduction in all-cause under-five mortality from 115 deaths per 1,000 in 2003 to 74 per 1,000 in 2008. In several sites where outpatient data on malaria have been monitored over several years, the number of clinical malaria cases has declined sharply. Similarly, on the coast of Kenya, hos-declined in the range of 28 to 63 percent over the period 1999–2007, while nonmalaria admissions were unchanged.[4]

  Progress has been achieved as a result of a comprehen-sive scale-up of malaria control and prevention measures, especially widespread distribution of ITNs, expanding and improving the IRS program, and increasing availability of effective antimalarial drugs. In conjunction with long-standing support by CDC for malaria research and policy development, USAID has supported malaria control efforts in Kenya for over a decade, including $5.5 million in FY 2006, $6 million in PMI jump start funding in FY 2007, $19.8 million in FY 2008, and $19.7 million in FY 2009.

Follow-up nationwide household surveys for the remaining nine PMI focus countries will be completed between 2010 and 2012 to contribute to the final assessment of pitalizations due to clinical malaria progress across all 15 PMI countries.

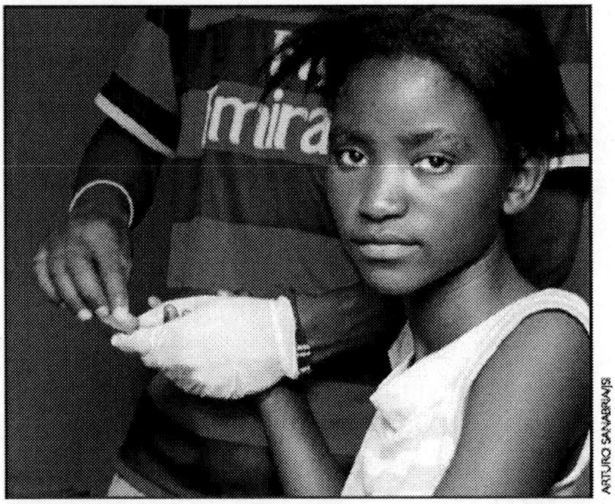

A young woman in the Kanyama Urban Health Center, Lusaka, Zambia, is tested for malaria with an RDT. With the scale-up of effective control measures, an increasing percentage of people with fever will not have malaria infections and will need to be correctly diagnosed and treated for other conditions.

Challenges and Future Directions

The work of PMI and other partners has already led to substantial reductions in malaria burden in six of the PMI focus countries. PMI, in collaboration with Roll Back Malaria partners, is beginning a comprehensive evaluation of how the scale-up of malaria control interventions has helped to reduce mortality in children under five years of age across Africa. The results of this evaluation will be available in early 2012. As part of this evaluation, PMI is also looking at the impact of malaria control efforts and the reduction in malaria morbidity and mortality on the health system as a whole.

For more in-depth information about PMI's monitoring and evaluation efforts, including the complete PMI monitoring and evaluation strategy document, please visit the monitoring and evaluation section of the PMI website at http://www.pmi.gov/technical/mne/index.html.

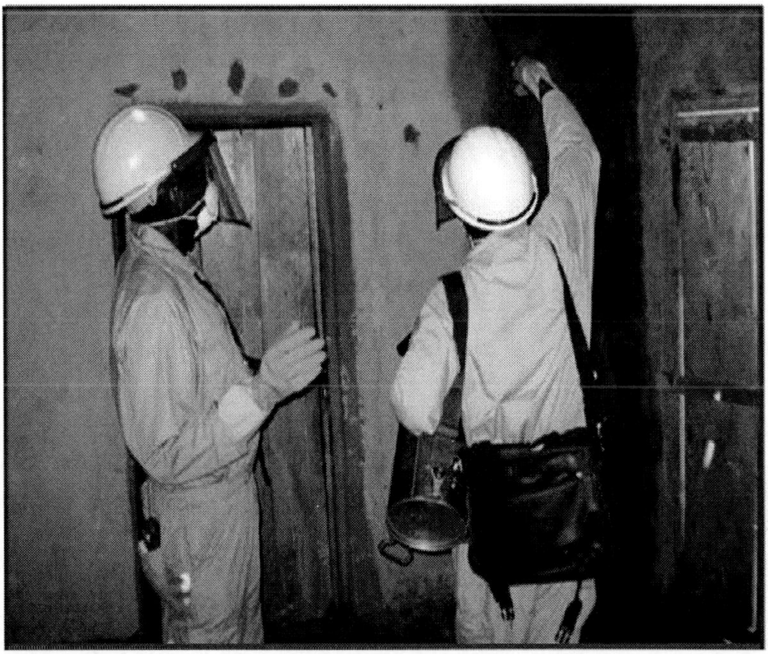

WAYNE STINSON/PMI

During an IRS campaign in Rwanda, a supervisor (left) provides guidance to a spray operator. Quality of spraying is essential for effective IRS, and frequent supervision ensures appropriate distribution of insecticide. PMI has raised awareness of the value and feasibility of IRS as a malaria control measure in Africa.

VOICES FROM THE FIELD

'Malaria Is No Longer Our Problem Here

The above is the sentiment of Chief Nurse Arona Guèye at the Kaymor Health Post in Senegal. Arona has been looking closely at the data from his rural health facility over the past three years, and he has seen a marked decline in the proportion of fever cases that are confirmed as malaria cases. In 2007, the year that both indoor residual spraying (IRS) and rapid diagnostic tests (RDTs) were introduced in his community, about 30 percent of the fever cases that he saw were malaria. During that time, he treated so many severe malaria cases that the health post was full, forcing him to treat some patients in his own home. In the most recent rainy season, however, he confirmed only 17 cases of malaria; none was severe, and nine of those were in residents from the nearby city of Kaolack. "I tell you," Arona comments, "it is clear now that IRS, combined with the ITNs we had already received, produced exceptional results. Malaria is backing down, and if this trend continues, the next generation of nurses will not be able to recognize a clinical severe malaria case."

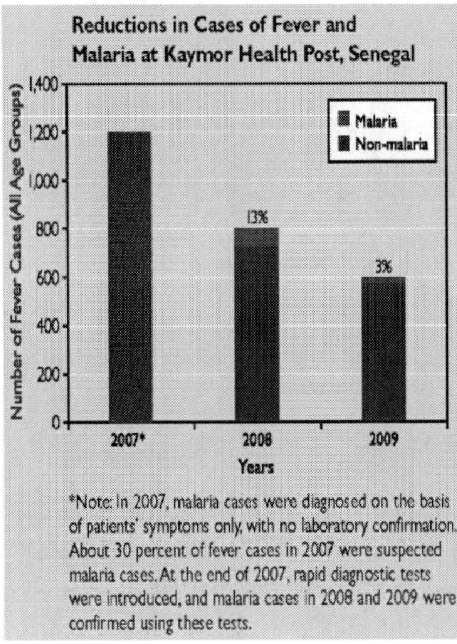

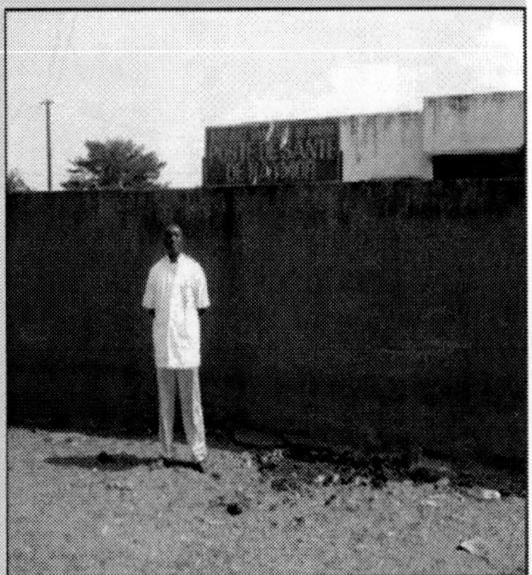

Chief Nurse Arona Guèye stands outside of the Kaymor Health Post in Senegal, where malaria cases have declined with the increase in malaria prevention activities.

8. U.S. GOVERNMENT MALARIA RESEARCH

"I am very pleased to see the donor community, host country governments, the private sector and foundations,such as the Bill and Melinda Gates Foundation and others, working together on a common target – endingmalaria deaths. We still have a long way to go. To accomplish this, we must continue to engage new partnersand support research and the technical partnerships that come in at every level."

– Rear Admiral R.T. Ziemer, USN (ret), U.S. Global Malaria Coordinator, October 1, 2009

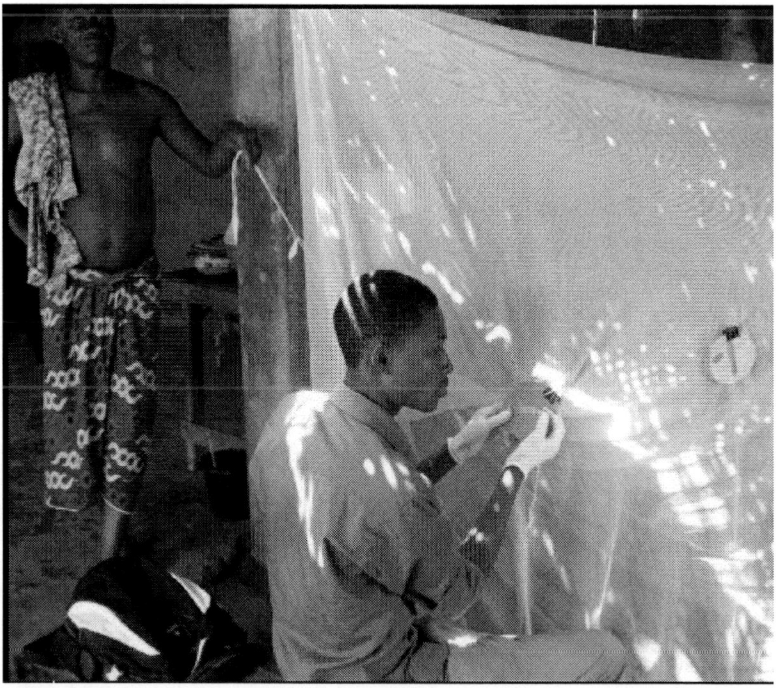

In Benin, a technician from the Centre de Recherche Entomologique de Cotonou (CREC) uses a rapid colorimetric field test tomeasure insecticide levels on an insecticide-treated net (ITN). In an operational research study, PMI partnered with CRECand successfully determined that the technology could be used to predict an ITN's efficacy over time. PMI plans to use thistechnology to help national malaria control programs determine net replacement need and to plan scale-up strategies.

The U.S. Government (USG) is committed to significantly reducing the global burden of malaria by supporting research through a coordinated and collaborative approach agencies and research partners around the globe. The USG malaria research portfolio involves USG agencies, such as the Centers for Disease Control and Prevention (CDC) and the National Institutes of Health (NIH) of the Department of Health and Human Services (HHS), the Walter Reed Army Institute of Research (WRAIR) and the Naval Medical Research Center (NMRC) of the Department of Defense, and USAID.

These USG agencies work with a wide range of partners that includes malaria-endemic country government agencies, private companies, universities, research institutes, and nongovernmental organizations. USG-supported malaria research has made contributions in the following areas:

- Defining of basic malaria biology and pathogenesis to design new interventions;
- Vaccine development and efficacy trials;
- Novel drug development to address resistance;
- Evaluating and setting of standards for diagnostic tests;
- Improved treatment strategies for severe malaria disease; and
- Operational research to improve project implementa-tion and impact.

The partnerships strengthen local capacity and contribute to the sustainability of national malaria control efforts. The USG is providing direction and momentum toward the ambitious goal of worldwide malaria control by ensuring that basic research and product development are effectively translated into field-applicable interventions that help reduce the burden of malaria.

PMI Operations Research Activities

An essential part of successful program planning and implementation is the capacity to determine current among intergovernmental priorities and best strategies, to ensure the quality of commodities or services, and to plan for challenges that will arise as malaria interventions are scaled up. For these reasons, PMI has supported operations research projects that are designed to improve program implementation as well as contribute to the global malaria control effort. PMI has prioritized research questions in collaboration with national malaria control programs (NMCPs) and, to avoid overlap, has coordinated with other organizations funding research (e.g., CDC, NIH, Bill and Melinda Gates Foundation, and The Global Fund to Fight AIDS, Tuberculosis and Malaria). Examples of ongoing studies address each of the key intervention areas within PMI:

- **Vector control (indoor residual spraying [IRS] and insecticide-treated nets [ITNs]):** Evaluating the longevity of commercially available ITNs, studying the combined use of different insecticide types to prevent the development of resistance, and measuring the combined use of both IRS and ITNs in different transmission settings;
- **Case management:** Developing a costed strategy for the introduction of treatment for severe malaria and other illnesses in children and

assessing the adequacy of the national diagnostics algorithm to ensure appro priate treatment of malaria; and

- Prevention of malaria in pregnancy: Evaluating the effectiveness of current national strategies using intermittent preventive treatment for pregnant women (IPTp) in the context of decreasing malaria transmission and increasing sulfadoxine-pyrimethamine (SP) resistance.

To date, more than 35 studies have been approved for support from PMI.

PMI-supported studies that have been completed have directly benefited malaria programs in the following ways: reduction of antimalarial drug use.

- An assessment in the city of Luanda, Angola, showed that malaria transmission was very low. As a result of these findings, the Angolan NMCP changed its malaria control strategy in Luanda to promote laboratory confirmation of malaria before treatment, and it has focused its malaria prevention efforts on the surrounding rural areas.
- A simple field-based test to assess the level of insecticide on ITNs was piloted and validated in Benin. The technology has been transferred to an in-country partner so that effectiveness of ITNs can be monitored as a quality assurance measure (see photo on page 53).
- A study of health workers in 20 clinics in Tanzania showed that introducing rapid diagnostic tests (RDTs) along with specific training in malaria case management resulted in improvements in prescribing practices of health workers with a 50 percent overall reduction of antimalarial drug use.

Most recently, in November 2009, PMI issued a request for applications to support field studies of the efficacy of combined and/or complementary use of IRS and ITNs in areas where malaria transmission has been reduced. In many countries, both long-lasting ITNs and IRS programs are being implemented in the same geographic areas, although little is known about how to optimize malaria control with a combination of these two inter-ventions. Results from these studies will help inform PMI programming across the 15 focus countries.

The development and execution of PMI-supported research projects involve the NMCPs and host country institutions. This approach fosters the development of in-country research capacity and collaboration between these entities. In turn, these partnerships and strengthened local capacity contribute to sustainable program management based on reliable local information.

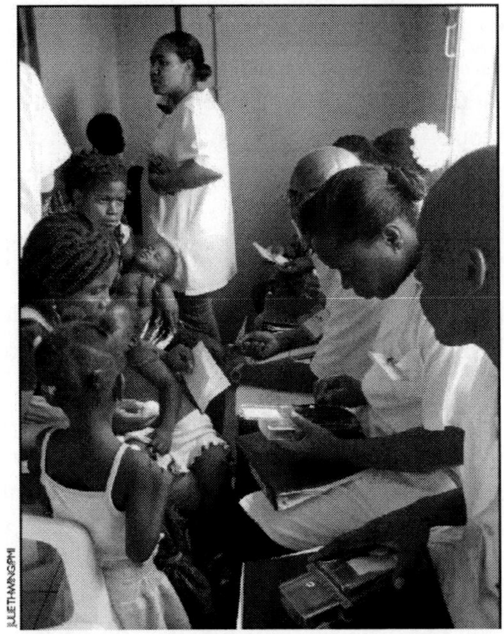

As part of a PMI operational research study, health workers test children with fever for malaria in a busy clinic in Luanda, the capital of Angola. The very low prevalence of malaria found in the city allowed the NMCP and PMI to focus malaria resources on rural areas, where the rates of malaria infection are higher.

Vaccine Development

USG supports the development and implementation of effective and safe malaria vaccines to add to the arsenal of malaria control interventions. Malaria vaccines may target three specific stages of the malaria parasite: sporozoites, to protect against infection by mosquitoes; blood stages, to reduce disease complications and deaths; and gametocytes, to prevent further transmission of parasites to mosquitoes.

The USAID Malaria Vaccine Development Program and the U.S. Military Malaria Vaccine Program: The mission of the USAID Malaria Vaccine Development Program (MVDP) is to develop vaccines as a part of control programs to reduce malaria mortality and morbidity in residents of endemic countries, especially children under five and pregnant women.

The U.S. Military Malaria Vaccine Program is a combined effort by WRAIR and the NMRC to develop vaccines to protect military personnel deployed in endemic areas.

Both of these programs have made major contributions to malaria vaccine development, including the support of seminal sporozoite studies that led to the development of the most advanced malaria vaccine to date – RTS,S – by WRAIR and GlaxoSmithKline. Over the past six years, several Phase I/II/IIb trials have shown the RTS,S vaccine to be a promising and safe vaccine, with a 50 percent protective efficacy in preventing severe malaria. Recent studies show that the vaccine can be safely co-administered with routine childhood vaccinations.

WRAIR and the CDC, collaborating partners in Kenya, are working with colleagues in seven African countries to conduct a large phase III trial of the RTS,S vaccine. The trial, sponsored by the Medical Vaccine Initiative, was initiated in 2009 and aims to enroll 16,000 children. If results continue to be promising, RTS,S could be the first malaria vaccine licensed and available for use.

While WRAIR is primarily focused on vaccines, like RTS,S, designed to stimulate antibody production, NMRC is focusing on vaccines that stimulate cellular immunity. Both have been shown to be important in the protective immune responses against malaria. These programs target the two species responsible for most malarial illnesses and deaths in the world: *Plasmodium falciparum*, the most lethal form of malaria, and *Plasmodium vivax*. During 2009, MVDP and the U.S. Military Malaria Vaccine Program showed that their *P? falciparum* blood-stage candidate vaccines, FMP2. 1/AS 02A provided protection against malaria University of Bamako in Mali and the Kenya Medical Research Institute. The MVDP supported a clinical trial of a vaccine regimen that provided evidence that cellular immunity can protect against malaria.

Drug Development

The USG focuses on drug development research, in con-cert with other global development efforts, to accelerate the availability of affordable and appropriate treatments for developing countries.

Medicines for Malaria Venture (MMV): MMV is a nonprofit, public-private partnership created in 1999 by the World Health Organization (WHO), the World Bank, and bilateral donor governments to replenish and sustain the global pipeline of antimalarial drugs. Its goal is to register at least one new antimalarial drug every five is on discovery and development of affordable to populations living in malaria-endemic areas.

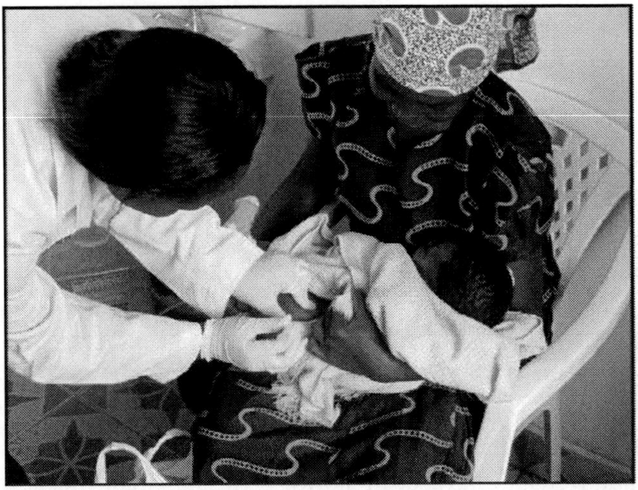
ALICE ONSASE AND KEVIN SHIKANGA KEMRI/CDC

Nurse Dinah Mauti Maragwa gives malaria candidate vaccine to an infant at the Siaya Kenya Medical Research Institute/CDC Malaria Vaccine Trial Site in Kenya. The U.S. Government supports the development and implementation of effective and safe malaria vaccines to add to the arsenal of malaria control interventions.

Since its inception, MMV has established more than 50 individual drug discovery and development projects, with emphasis on those that are effective against drug-based resistant strains of *P. falciparum*, particularly those projects that can be used safely in young children and pregnant women. The research and development activities are carried out at a broad variety of institutions, comprising more than 40 academic and pharmaceutical and FMP0 10/AS 0 1B, organizations located in 10 different countries, including in trials with the the United States. In December 2008, dispersible artemether-lumefantrine became the first MMV-supported antimalarial drug to receive strict regulatory authority approval; it has since been approved for use in 21 countries. The dossier for dihydroartemisinin-piperaquine has been submitted to the European Medicines Agency. In addition, a dossier is being prepared for pyronaridine-artesunate after the completion of Phase III trials.

Walter Reed Army Institute of Research Drug Development Program: WRAIR manages a comprehensive program of antimalarial drug development. WRAIR's mission is to develop new prophylactic drugs as well as drugs that can eliminate the latent liver stages of *P.vivax*. In collaboration with the pharmaceutical industry, WRAIR was instrumental in the development and approval of mefloquine and doxycycline, two of the three years. MMV's focus drugs that are currently approved for malaria prevention. drugs that will be

WHO Special Programme for Research and Training in Tropical Diseases (WHO/TDR): WHO/TDR has support from USAID for multiyear studies in three areas:

- To demonstrate the relative safety of artemisinin-based combination therapies (ACTs) in the second and third trimesters of pregnancy and a pilot study of enhanced pharmacovigilance;
- To assess the effectiveness of integrating community- based malaria case management with pneumonia and diarrhea (two other major killers of children under five); and
- To assess the use of RDTs in the case management of malaria at the community level.

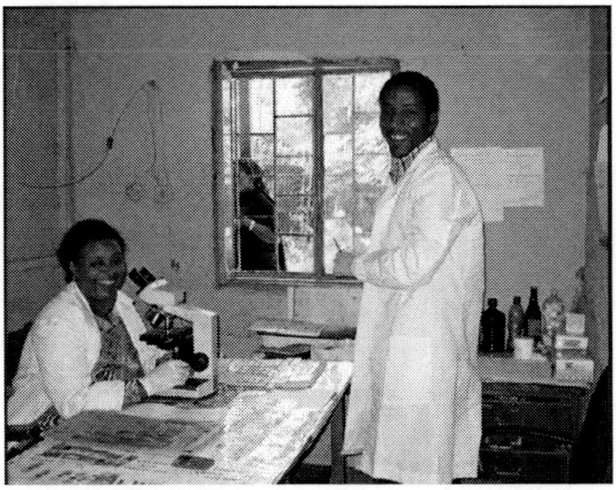

Two laboratory technicians collect, stain, and read blood films to confirm malaria diagnoses at Bishoftu Malaria Center, Ethiopia. Patients who were identified to have malaria parasites were assessed by a clinical team for enrollment in a therapeutic efficacy study against the national first-line treatments.

USG Malaria Research Organizations

The CDC and the National Institute of Allergy and Infectious Diseases (NIAID) have well known comprehensive malaria research programs that conduct basic research to develop and test new malaria interventions as well as provide expertise to improve malaria control efforts around the globe.

CDC Malaria Branch: In addition to applied research within PMI and USAID's regional initiatives for the Amazon and Mekong Basin countries, CDC investiga-tors are engaged in a broad range of research activities with the objectives of:

- Identifying new antimalarial drug compounds and vaccine candidates and evaluating their potential efficacy in nonhuman primates;
- Evaluating new tools for malaria diagnosis, treatment, and for ensuring their quality;
- Establishing the optimal mix of malaria control inter-ventions in different malaria transmission settings; and
- Exploring opportunities to integrate malaria inter- ventions and their monitoring into other health and development initiatives in endemic countries.

CDC investigators provide expertise to global malaria research consortia, including those focusing on ACTs, health systems, malaria elimination/ eradication, malaria in pregnancy, malaria transmission, and malaria vaccines. taken leadership roles in:

- Studying the burden and treatment options for malaria in pregnancy;
- Evaluating the efficacy of a promising malaria vaccine candidate;
- Assessing the efficacy of new insecticide-treated materials;
- Monitoring the quality of commercially available diagnostic tests for malaria and malaria treatment drugs; and
- Monitoring the effectiveness and cost-effectiveness of strategies to enhance the availability of malaria treatment.

National Institute of Allergy and Infectious Diseases and prevention (NIAID): NIAID, which has a long-standing interest in global health, is the lead USG agency in malaria research. To accomplish its goal of reducing morbidity and mortality from malaria, NIAID focuses on:

- Understanding the biology of malaria parasites and their interactions with mosquito vectors and human hosts, including conducting genomic research;
- Developing tools for effective and sustainable malaria prevention, treatment, and control;
- Enhancing research infrastructure, including clinical CDC scientists have research, in malaria-endemic countries; and
- Encouraging global cooperation in malaria research.

NIAID researchers study the biology of malaria parasites and mosquito vectors, as well as disease pathogenesis and immunology, characterizing the mechanisms by which and by which malaria parasites infect and survive in the human host and by which infection results in disease. Understanding these mechanisms should yield new approaches to prevention and treatment. NIAID has worked in the following areas:

- Genomics: Supplying scientists with the complete genetic sequences of the mosquito vector *Anopheles gambiae* and the parasites *P. falciparum* and *P. vivax* to help identify new targets for effective disease interventions such as vaccines or drugs.
- Vaccine development: Identifying novel vaccine candidates by characterizing protective immunological responses to malaria parasites from various life cycle stages, which could confer protection from infection or disease. Alternative strategies seek to identify transmission-blocking vaccines that will prevent transmission to the mosquito vector.
- Drug development: Developing new methods and improving existing ones for the treatment of malaria, including the identification and characterization of unique parasite biochemical pathways that may serve as targets for drugs; determination of mode of action of existing and potential drugs; and analysis of themechanisms of drug resistance.
- Diagnostics: Developing easy-to-use tests for the diagnosis of malaria infections and the identification of parasite drug-resistance profiles.
- Clinical research: Strengthening field site capacity for research and clinical trials on drugs, vaccines, and diagnostics and supporting multiple vaccine clinical trials in the United States and in malaria-endemic countries. NIAID also seeks to expand research in different geographic areas and epidemiologic settings, in susceptible

populations (such as infants, young children, and pregnant women), and in individuals with different clinical manifestations.

NIAID also invests heavily in developing and strengthening sustainable local research capacity in disease-endemic countries. To assist capacity strengthening, NIAID provides scientists working in the United States and in malaria-endemic countries access to critical malaria research resources and, working with the Fogarty International Center at NIH, helps train and educate **new** investigators in the field.

ACKNOWLEDGMENTS

The Fourth Annual Report of the President's Malaria Initiative is dedicated to the staff of host governments, international and local partners, and all U.S. Government staff who have contributed to the achievements described in these pages.

End Notes

[1] Rowe, A., et al. 2007. Evaluating the impact of malaria control efforts on mortality in sub-Saharan Africa. *Tropical Medicine and International Health*, 12 (12): 1524–1539.

[2] National Malaria Control Programme. 2009. Summary of Five Household Surveys to Monitor Population-level Coverage and Impact of Malaria Interventions in Tanzania, 2007–08. Dar es Salaam, Tanzania.

[3] Smithson, P. 2009. Down but not out: The impact of malaria control in Tanzania. Spotlight Issue 2 (May 2009), Ifakara Health Institute, 8pp.

[4] Okiro EA, Hay SI, Gikandi PW, Sharif SK, Noor AM, Peshu N, Marsk K, Snow RW. 2007. The decline in pediatric malaria admissions on the Coast of Kenya *Malaria Journal*, 6: 151.

APPENDIX 1. PMI FUNDING FY 2006–FY 2010

PMI FUNDING								
	PMI Focus Country Programs	FY 2005 Jump Start Funding	FY 2006	FY 2007[1]	FY 2008[2]	FY 2009	FY 2010 Preliminary3	Total
Round 1 Countries	Angola	1,740,000	7,500,000	18,500,000	18,846,000	18,700,000	35,500,000	
	Tanzania	2,000,000	11,500,000	31,000,000	33,725,000	35,000,000	52,000,000	
	Uganda	510,775	9,500,000	21,500,000	21,822,000	21,600,000	35,000,000	
Round 2 Countries	Malawi	-	2,045,000	18,500,000	17,854,000	17,700,000	27,000,000	
	Mozambique	-	6,259,000	18,000,000	19,838,000	19,700,000	38,000,000	
	Rwanda	-	1,479,000	20,000,000	16,862,000	16,300,000	18,000,000	
	Senegal	-	2,168,000	16,700,000	15,870,000	15,700,000	27,000,000	
Round 3 Countries	Benin	-	1,774,000	3,600,000	13,887,000	13,800,000	21,000,000	
	Ethiopia	-	2,563,000	6,700,000	19,838,000	19,700,000	31,000,000	
	Ghana	-	1,478,000	5,000,000	16,862,000	17,300,000	34,000,000	
	Kenya	-	5,470,000	6,050,000	19,838,000	19,700,000	40,000,000	
	Liberia	-	-	2,500,000	12,399,000	11,800,000	18,000,000	
	Madagascar	-	2,169,000	5,000,000	16,862,000	16,700,000	33,900,000	
	Mali	-	2,490,000	4,500,000	14,879,000	15,400,000	28,000,000	
	Zambia	-	7,659,000	9,470,000	14,879,000	14,700,000	25,600,000	
	Headquarters	-	1,500,000	10,000,000	21,596,500	26,100,000	36,000,000	
	PMI TOTAL	-	**30,000,000**	**154,200,000**	**295,857,500**	**299,900,000**	**500,000,000**	**1,279,957,500**
	JUMP START TOTAL	**4,250,775**	**35,554,000**	**42,820,000**				
	TOTAL	**4,250,775**	**65,554,000**	**197,020,000**	**295,857,500**	**299,900,000**	**500,000,000**	

[1] $25 million plus-up funds include $22 million allocated to 15 PMI countries ($19.2 million for Round 2 countries and $2.8 million for jump starts in Round 3 countries).

[2] Levels after Agency 0.081% recession.

[3] Preliminary allocations subject to final approval by the Coordinator and final appropriations.

APPENDIX 2. PMI ACTIVITY SUMMARY

1. Indoor Residual Spraying

RESIDENTS PROTECTED BY PMI-SUPPORTED INDOOR RESIDUAL SPRAYING[1,2]					
	Country	**PMIYear[1] (2006)**	**PMIYear[2] (2007)**	**PMIYear[3] (2008)**	**PMIYear[4] (2009)**
Round 1 Countries	Angola	590,398	612,776	992,856	485,974
	Tanzania	1,018,156	1,279,960	1,569,071	2,087,062
	Uganda	488,502	1,865,956	2,211,388	2,262,578
Round 2 Countries	Malawi	-	126,126	106,450	299,744
	Mozambique	-	2,593,949	1,457,142	2,263,409
	Rwanda	-	720,764	885,957	1,329,340
	Senegal	-	678,971	645,346	661,814
Round 3 Countries	Benin	-	-	521,738	512,491
	Ethiopia	-	3,890,000	5,921,906	6,484,297
	Ghana	-	-	601,973	708,103
	Kenya	-	3,459,207	3,061,967	1,435,272
	Liberia	-	-	-	163,149
	Madagascar	-	-	2,561,034	1,274,809
	Mali	-	-	420,580	497,122
	Zambia	-	3,600,000	4,200,000	6,500,000
	TOTAL	**2,097,056**	**18,827,709**	**25,157,408**	**26,965,164**

(Continued)

HOUSES SPRAYED WITH PMI SUPPORT[3,4]					
	Country	**PMIYear1 (2006)**	**PMIYear2 (2007)**	**PMIYear3 (2008)**	**PMIYear4 (2009)**
Round 1 Countries	Angola	107,373	110,826	189,259	102,73 1
	Tanzania	203,754	247,712	308,058	422,749
	Uganda	103,329	446,117	575,903	567,035
Round 2 Countries	Malawi	-	26,950	24,764	74,772
	Mozambique	-	586,568	412,923	571,194
	Rwanda	-	159,063	189,756	295,174
	Senegal	-	169,743	153,942	176,279
Round 3 Countries	Benin	-	-	142,814	156,223
	Ethiopia	-	778,000	1,793,248	1,935,402
	Ghana	-	-	254,305	284,856
	Kenya	-	1,171,073	764,050	517,051
	Liberia	-	-	-	20,400
	Madagascar	-	-	422,132	216,060
	Mali	-	-	107,638	126,922
	Zambia	-	657,695	762,479	1,189,676
	TOTAL	**414,456**	**4,353,747**	**6,101,271**	**6,656,524**
SPRAY PERSONNEL TRAINED WITH PMI SUPPORT[5,6]					
Round 1 Countries	Angola	350	582	2,104	585
	Tanzania	536	734	688	2,806
	Uganda	450	4,062	4,945	4,412

(Continued)

	Country	PMIYear1 (2006)	PMIYear2 (2007)	PMIYear3 (2008)	PMIYear4 (2009)
Round 2 Countries	Malawi	-	300	309	462
	Mozambique	-	1,190	1,282	1,343
	Rwanda	-	655	2,091	2,276
	Senegal	-	275	706	570
Round 3 Countries	Benin	-	-	335	347
	Ethiopia	-	-	1,198	3,017
	Ghana	-	-	468	577
	Kenya	-	4,697	1,452	1,719
	Liberia	-	-	-	340
	Madagascar	-	-	1,673	851
	Mali	-	-	413	424
	Zambia	-	1,300	1,413	1,935
	TOTAL	**1,336**	**13,795**	**19,077**	**21,664**

[1] A cumulative count of the number of people protected for Years 1 through 4 of PMI is not provided since some areas have been sprayed on more than one occasion.

[2] During 2009, the USG also provided support for an IRS campaign in Zimbabwe, which protected 929,600 people.

[3] A cumulative count of the number of houses sprayed for Years 1 through 4 of PMI is not provided since some areas have been sprayedon more than one occasion.

[4] During 2009, more than 600,000 structures were also sprayed in Zimbabwe with USG support.

[5] A cumulative count of the number of spray personnel trained for Years 1 through 4 of PMI is not provided since some personnel have beentrained on more than one occasion.

[6] Spray personnel are defined as spray operators, supervisors, and ancillary personnel. These calculations do not include many people trained toconduct information and community mobilization programs surrounding IRS campaigns.

2. Insecticide-Treated Nets

INSECTICIDE-TREATED NETS (ITNs) PROCURED AND DISTRIBUTED WITH PMI SUPPORT[1]						
		ITNs Procured ITNs Distributed				
	Country	PMIYear [1] (2006)	PMIYear [2] (2007)	PMIYear [3] (2008)	PMIYear [4] (2009)	Cumulative
Round 1 Countries	Angola	540,949	294,200	734,198	395,748	1,965,095
		540,949	-	339,440	446,348	1,326,737
	Tanzania	130,000	-	143,560	1,468,966	1,742,526
		130,000	-	113,560	1,498,966	1,742,526
	Uganda	376,444	1,132,532	480,000	765,940	2,754,916
		305,305	683,777	999,894	651,203	2,640,179
Round 2 Countries	Malawi	-	1,039,400	849,578	1,791,506	3,680,484
		-	211,995	849,578	851,436	1,913,009
	Mozambique	-	786,000	720,000	1,450,000	2,956,000
		-	565,000	842,802	930,000	2,337,802
	Rwanda	-	-	550,000	912,400	1,462,400
		-	-	-	500,000	500,000
	Senegal	-	200,000	790,000	408,000	1,398,000
		-	196,872	792,951	380,000	1,369,823
Round 3 Countries	Benin	-	221,000	385,697	875,000	1,481,697
		-	215,627	45,840	879,415	1,140,882
	Ethiopia	-	102,145	22,284	1,559,500	1,683,929
		-	102,145	22,284	559,500	683,929

(Continued)

	Country	PMIYear [1] (2006)	PMIYear [2] (2007)	PMIYear [3] (2008)	PMIYear [4] (2009)	Cumulative
	Ghana	-	60,023	350,000	955,000	1,365,023
		-	60,023	-	350,000	410,023
	Kenya	-	-	60,000	1,240,000	1,300,000
		-	-	60,000	550,000	610,000
	Liberia	-	197,000	-	430,000	627,000
		-	-	184,000	430,000	614,000
	Madagascar	-	-	351,900	1,805,007	2,156,907
		-	-	351,900	1,005,007	1,356,907
	Mali	-	369,800	858,060	600,000	1,827,860
		-	369,800	258,060	600,000	1,227,860
	Zambia	-	808,332	186,550	433,235	1,428,117
		-	550,017	444,865	433,235	1,428,117
	TOTAL	**1,047,393**	**5,210,432**	**6,481,827**	**15,090,302**	**27,829,954**
		976,254	**2,955,256**	**5,305,174**	**10,065,110**	**19,301,794**
INSECTICIDE-TREATED NETS PROCURED BY OTHER DONORS AND DISTRIBUTED WITH PMI SUPPORT						
Round 1 Countries	Angola	-	-	109,624	17,089	126,713
	Tanzania	-	-	350,000	117,400	467,400
	Uganda	-	369,900	-	-	369,900
Round 2 Countries	Malawi	-	-	-	10,700	10,700
	Mozambique	-	-	78,000	179,730	257,730
	Senegal	-	-	-	1,875,456	1,875,456

(Continued)

	Country	PMIYear [1] (2006)	PMIYear [2] (2007)	PMIYear [3] (2008)	PMIYear [4] (2009)	Cumulative
Round 3 Countries	Ethiopia	-	-	-	475,000	475,000
	Ghana	-	-	750,000	-	750,000
	Madagascar	-	-	-	290,636	290,636
	TOTAL	**-**	**369,900**	**1,287,624**	**2,966,0 1 1**	**4,623,535**
INSECTICIDE-TREATED NETS SOLD WITH PMI MARKETING SUPPORT						
Round 1 Countries	Uganda	586,284	932,033	1,1 15,074	281,955	2,915,346
Round 2 Countries	Senegal	-	158,060	57,832	57,929	273,821
Round 3 Countries	Ghana	-	612,000	1,234,159	347,520	2,193,679
	TOTAL	**586,284**	**1,702,093**	**2,407,065**	**687,404**	**5,382,846**
INSECTICIDE-TREATED NETS REDEEMED THROUGH VOUCHER PROGRAMS WITH PMI SUPPORT						
Round 1 Countries	Tanzania	-	362,194	1,034,711	596,275	1,993,180
Round 2 Countries	Senegal	-	134,413	168,206	72,234	374,853
Round 3 Countries	Ghana	-	-	236,789	102,833	339,622
	TOTAL	**-**	**496,607**	**1,439,706**	**771,342**	**2,707,655**

[1] During 2009, the USG also provided support for ITN activities in the Democratic Republic of the Congo, Nigeria, and Sudan; more than 852,000 ITNs were procured and distributed.

3. Malaria in Pregnancy

SULFADOXINE-PYRIMETHAMINE (SP) TREATMENTS PROCURED AND DISTRIBUTED WITH PMI SUPPORT[1]						
		SP Treatments Procured				
		SP Treatments Distributed				
	Country	PMIYear 1 (2006)	PMIYear 2 (2007)	PMIYear 3 (2008)	PMIYear 4 (2009)	Cumulative
Round 1 Countries	Uganda	-	-	18,333	72,666	90,999
		-	-	2,556	45,780	48,336
Round 2 Countries	Rwanda	-	583,333	-	-	583,333
		-	583,333	-	-	583,333
Round 3 Countries	Benin	-	766,666	-	-	766,666
		-	-	-	307,121	307,121
	Kenya	-	-	-	840,000	840,000
		-	-	-	840,000	840,000
	Liberia	-	-	-	78,666	78,666
		-	-	-	78,666	78,666
	Mali	-	-	1,000,000	-	1,000,000
		-	-	-	1,000,000	1,000,000
	Zambia	-	-	-	666,666	666,666
		-	-	-	666,666	666,666
	TOTAL	-	**1,349,999**	**1,018,333**	**1,657,998**	**4,026,330**
		-	**583,333**	**2,556**	**2,938,233**	**3,524,122**

(Continued)

HEALTH WORKERS TRAINED IN IPTp USE WITH PMI SUPPORT [3,4]						
	Country	**PMIYear 1 (2006)**	**PMIYear 2 (2007)**	**PMIYear 3 (2008)**	**PMIYear 4 (2009)**	**Cumulative**
Round 1 Countries	Angola	1,450	290	1,481	2,554	
	Tanzania	376	1,158	2,532	2,288	
	Uganda	168	807	649	724	
Round 2 Countries	Malawi	-	-	2,747	348	
	Rwanda	-	250	436	-	
	Senegal	-	43	2,422	865	
Round 3 Countries	Benin	-	605	1,267	146	
	Ghana	-	-	464	1,170	
	Kenya	-	-	-	5,107	
	Liberia	-	-	417	750	
	Mali	-	-	142	-	
	Zambia	-	-	-	63	
	TOTAL	1,994	3,153	12,557	14,015	

[1] During 2009, the USG also provided support for malaria in pregnancy activities in the Democratic Republic of the Congo, Nigeria, and Sudan; 430,000 SP treatments were procured and distributed.

[2] During 2009, the USG also provided support for malaria in pregnancy activities in the Democratic Republic of the Congo, Nigeria, andSudan; more than 700 health workers were trained in IPTp.

[3] A cumulative count of individual health workers trained is not provided since some health workers have been trained on more than one occasion.

4. Case Management

ARTEMISININ-BASED COMBINATION THERAPY (ACT) PROCURED AND DISTRIBUTED WITH PMI SUPPORT[1]						
		ACTs Procured				
		ACTs Distributed				
	Country	PMIYear 1 (2006)	PMIYear 2 (2007)	PMIYear 3 (2008)	PMIYear 4 (2009)	Cumulative
Round 1 Countries	Angola	587,520	2,033,200	3,035,520	5,572,860	11,229,100
		-	1,689,321	3,109,089	1,947,188	6,745,598
	Tanzania	380,160	694,050	146,730	4,001,880	5,222,820
		380,160	494,050	346,730	544,017	1,764,957
	Uganda	261,870	-	1,140,480	-	1,402,350
		227,827	-	-	1,140,480	1,368,307
Round 2 Countries	Malawi	-	4,694,013	4,501,740	5,139,600	14,335,353
		-	4,694,013	3,579,278	3,693,510	11,966,801
	Mozambique	-	1,440,000	3,525,120	3,549,758	8,514,878
		-	220,230	1,440,000	2,210,320	3,870,550
	Rwanda	-	715,000	-	-	715,000
		-	-	715,000	-	715,000
	Senegal	-	-	-	444,420	444,420
		-	-	-	-	-
Round 3 Countries	Benin	-	1,465,170	-	215,100	1,680,270
		-	153,884	326,544	812,232	1,292,660
	Ethiopia	-	-	600,000	1,081,000	1,681,000
		-	-	-	1,681,000	1,681,000
	Ghana	-	1,142,759	-	1,142,759	
		-	-	1,028,000	1,028,000	

(Continued)

	Country	PMIYear 1 (2006)	PMIYear 2 (2007)	PMIYear 3 (2008)	PMIYear 4 (2009)	Cumulative
	Kenya	-	-	1,281,720	7,804,800	9,086,520
		-	-	1,281,720	6,015,360	7,297,080
	Liberia	-	496,000	-	1,303,175	1,799,175
		-	-	496,000	1,303,175	1,799,175
	Madagascar	-	-	-	-	-
		-	-	-	-	-
	Mali	-	-	-	330,589	330,589
		-	-	-	330,589	330,589
	Zambia	-	-	80,640	173,160	253,800
		-	-	80,640	173,160	253,800
	TOTAL	1,229,550	11,537,433	15,454,709	29,616,342	57,838,034
		607,987	7,251,498	11,375,001	20,879,031	40,113,517

[1] During 2009, the USG also provided support for case management activities in the Democratic Republic of the Congo, Nigeria, and Sudan; more than 6.2 million ACTs were procured, of which 5.4 million were distributed.

ACTs PROCURED BY OTHER DONORS AND DISTRIBUTED WITH PMI SUPPORT						
	Country	**PMIYear1 (2006)**	**PMIYear2 (2007)**	**PMIYear3 (2008)**	**PMIYear4 (2009)**	**Cumulative**
Round 1 Countries	Uganda	-	8,709,140	112,330	4,459,918	13,281,388
Round 2 Countries	Malawi	-	-	-	2,056,170	2,056,170
	Mozambique	-	-	-	1,423,350	1,423,350
	Rwanda	-	-	-	396,625	396,625
Round 3 Countries	Madagascar	-	-	-	519,338	519,338
	TOTAL	-	**8,709,140**	**112,330**	**8,855,401**	**17,676,871**

HEALTH WORKERS TRAINED IN ACT USE WITH PMI SUPPORT [1,2]					
	Country	**PMIYear 1 (2006)**	**PMIYear2 (2007)**	**PMIYear3 (2008)**	**PMIYear4 (2009)**
Round 1 Countries	Angola	1,283	290	1,357	2,784
	Tanzania	4,217	1,011	1,767	1,018
	Uganda	2,844	12,637	9,159	1,356
Round 2 Countries	Malawi	-	-	5,315	809
	Mozambique	-	174	422	16,768
	Rwanda	-	5,127	8,565	7,672
	Senegal	-	1,020	4,776	1,162
Round 3 Countries	Benin	-	605	-	762
	Ethiopia	-	-	2,786	-
	Ghana	-	-	368	1,144
	Kenya	-	-	-	4,747
	Liberia	-	-	595	746
	Madagascar	-	-	-	1,696
	Mali	-	-	101	412
	Zambia	-	-	186	197
	TOTAL	**8,344**	**20,864**	**35,397**	**41,273**

[1] During 2009, the USG also provided support for case management activities in the Democratic Republic of the Congo, Nigeria, and Sudan; more than 3,000 health workers were trained in the use of ACTs.

[2] A cumulative count of individual health workers trained for Years 1 through 4 of PMI is not provided since some health workers have been trained on more than one occasion.

RAPID DIAGNOSTIC TESTS (RDTs) PROCURED AND DISTRIBUTED WITH PMI SUPPORT						
		RDTs Procured RDTs Distributed				
	Country	PMIYear 1 (2006)	PMIYear 2 (2007)	PMIYear 3 (2008)	PMIYear 4 (2009)	Cumulative
Round 1 Countries	Angola	129,875	375,000	375,000	600,000	1,479,875
		-	101,000	380,875	975,000	1,456,875
	Tanzania	875,000	550,200	1,075,000	950,000	3,450,200
		250,000	1,025,200	425,000	989,500	2,689,700
Round 3 Countries	Benin	-	178,400	-	-	178,400
		-	73,815	104,585	-	178,400
	Ethiopia	-	-	-	1,640,000	1,640,000
		-	-	-	820,000	820,000
	Ghana	-	-	-	1,850	1,850
		-	-	-	1,850	1,850
	Liberia	-	-	-	850,000	850,000
		-	-	-	850,000	850,000
	Mali	-	-	-	41,500	41,500
		-	-	-	14,000	14,000
	Zambia	-	979,000	660,000	2,070,000	3,709,000
		-	-	979,000	1,250,000	2,229,000
	TOTAL	**1,004,875**	**2,082,600**	**2,110,000**	**6,153,350**	**11,350,825**
		250,000	**1,200,015**	**1,889,460**	**4,900,350**	**8,239,825**

HEALTH WORKERS TRAINED IN MALARIA DIAGNOSIS WITH PMI SUPPORT[1]

	Country	PMIYear1 (2006)	PMIYear2 (2007)	PMIYear3 (2008)	PMIYear4 (2009)
Round 1 Countries	Angola	-	374	1,356	691
	Tanzania	-	-	-	247
	Uganda	-	-	100	1,115
Round 2 Countries	Mozambique	-	391	-	136
	Senegal	-	-	90	19
Round 3 Countries	Benin	-	605	-	24
	Ghana	-	-	-	46
	Kenya	-	-	77	-
	Liberia	-	-	-	22
	Madagascar	-	-	-	108
	Mali	-	-	40	412
	Zambia	-	-	-	36
	TOTAL	**-**	**1,370**	**1,663**	**2,856**

[1] A cumulative count of individual health workers trained for Years 1 through 4 of PMI is not provided since some have been trained on more than one occasion.

APPENDIX 3. PMI COUNTRY-LEVEL TARGETS

PMI has a single set of country-level targets for the four major control measures, which are the same for each focus country:

- More than 90 percent of households with a pregnant woman and/or children under five will own at least one ITN;
- 85 percent of children under five will have slept under an ITN the previous night;
- 85 percent of pregnant women will have slept under an ITN the previous night;
- 85 percent of houses in geographic areas targeted for IRS will have been sprayed;
- 85 percent of pregnant women and children under five will have slept under an ITN the previous night or in a house that has been protected by IRS;
- 85 percent of women who have completed a pregnancy in the last two years will have received two or more doses of IPTp during that pregnancy;
- 85 percent of governmental health facilities will have ACTs available for treatment of uncomplicated malaria; and
- 85 percent of children under five with suspected malaria will have received ACT treatment within 24 hours of onset of symptoms.[1]

[1] PMI is working with the Monitoring and Evaluation Reference Group of the Roll Back Malaria Partnership to develop a more effective indicator that captures effective case management of malaria. As control measures in many sub-Saharan African countries have been scaled up, the burden of malaria has been reduced, and an increasing proportion of fever illnesses are no longer caused by malaria. Therefore, giving malaria treatment based solely on the presence of fever is no longer an acceptable practice. This indicator thus needs to be reformulated as it no longer captures appropriate care seeking and treatment of malaria.

INDEX

C

D

E

F

G

M

N

O

U

V

W

Y

Z